THE SENSITIVE SKIN

Treatment Modalities and Cosmeceuticals

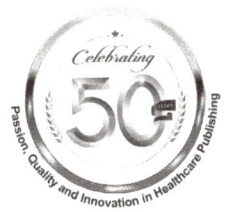

THE SENSITIVE SKIN

Treatment Modalities and Cosmeceuticals

Editors

Rashmi Sarkar MD MNAMS
Professor, Department of Dermatology
Maulana Azad Medical College and Lok Nayak Hospital
New Delhi, India

Surabhi Sinha MD DNB MNAMS
Specialist, Department of Dermatology and STD
Dr Ram Manohar Lohia Hospital and
Post Graduate Institute of Medical
Education and Research
New Delhi, India

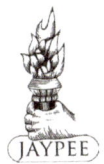

JAYPEE BROTHERS MEDICAL PUBLISHERS
The Health Sciences Publisher
New Delhi | London | Panama

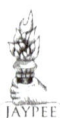

Jaypee Brothers Medical Publishers (P) Ltd

Headquarters

Jaypee Brothers Medical Publishers (P) Ltd
4838/24, Ansari Road, Daryaganj
New Delhi 110 002, India
Phone: +91-11-43574357
Fax: +91-11-43574314
Email: jaypee@jaypeebrothers.com

Overseas Offices

J.P. Medical Ltd
83 Victoria Street, London
SW1H 0HW (UK)
Phone: +44 20 3170 8910
Fax: +44 (0)20 3008 6180
Email: info@jpmedpub.com

Jaypee-Highlights Medical Publishers Inc
City of Knowledge, Bld. 235, 2nd Floor, Clayton
Panama City, Panama
Phone: +1 507-301-0496
Fax: +1 507-301-0499
Email: cservice@jphmedical.com

Jaypee Brothers Medical Publishers (P) Ltd
Bhotahity, Kathmandu, Nepal
Phone: +977-9741283608
Email: kathmandu@jaypeebrothers.com

Website: www.jaypeebrothers.com
Website: www.jaypeedigital.com

© 2019, Jaypee Brothers Medical Publishers

The views and opinions expressed in this book are solely those of the original contributor(s)/author(s) and do not necessarily represent those of editor(s) of the book.

All rights reserved. No part of this publication may be reproduced, stored or transmitted in any form or by any means, electronic, mechanical, photocopying, recording or otherwise, without the prior permission in writing of the publishers.

All brand names and product names used in this book are trade names, service marks, trademarks or registered trademarks of their respective owners. The publisher is not associated with any product or vendor mentioned in this book.

Medical knowledge and practice change constantly. This book is designed to provide accurate, authoritative information about the subject matter in question. However, readers are advised to check the most current information available on procedures included and check information from the manufacturer of each product to be administered, to verify the recommended dose, formula, method and duration of administration, adverse effects and contraindications. It is the responsibility of the practitioner to take all appropriate safety precautions. Neither the publisher nor the author(s)/editor(s) assume any liability for any injury and/or damage to persons or property arising from or related to use of material in this book.

This book is sold on the understanding that the publisher is not engaged in providing professional medical services. If such advice or services are required, the services of a competent medical professional should be sought.

Every effort has been made where necessary to contact holders of copyright to obtain permission to reproduce copyright material. If any have been inadvertently overlooked, the publisher will be pleased to make the necessary arrangements at the first opportunity. The **CD/DVD-ROM** (if any) provided in the sealed envelope with this book is complimentary and free of cost. **Not meant for sale.**

Inquiries for bulk sales may be solicited at: jaypee@jaypeebrothers.com

The Sensitive Skin: Treatment Modalities and Cosmeceuticals / Rashmi Sarkar, Surabhi Sinha

First Edition: **2019**

ISBN: 978-93-5270-544-3

Printed at

CONTRIBUTORS

EDITORS

Rashmi Sarkar MD MNAMS
Professor, Department of Dermatology
Maulana Azad Medical College and Lok Nayak Hospital
New Delhi, India

Surabhi Sinha MD DNB MNAMS
Specialist, Department of Dermatology and STD
Dr Ram Manohar Lohia Hospital and Post Graduate Institute of Medical Education and Research
New Delhi, India

CONTRIBUTING AUTHORS

Akreti S Sobti DDVL DNB
Specialist Dermatologist
Department of Dermatology
Minal Medical Centre
Dubai, UAE

Alireza Firooz MD
Professor
Department of Dermatology
Center for Research and Training in Skin Diseases and Leprosy
Tehran University of Medical Sciences
Tehran, Iran

Ambika Damodaran MD
Department of Dermatology
University of Michigan
Ann Arbor, Michigan, USA

Azin Ayatollahi MD
Assistant Professor
Department of Dermatology
Center for Research and Training in Skin Diseases and Leprosy
Tehran University of Medical Sciences
Tehran, Iran

Divya Arora MD DNB
Assistant Professor
Department of Dermatology
Subharti Medical College
Meerut, Uttar Pradesh, India

Indrashis Podder MD DNB
RMO cum Clinical Tutor
Department of Dermatology
College of Medicine and Sagore Dutta Hospital
Kolkata, West Bengal, India

The Sensitive Skin: Treatment Modalities and Cosmeceuticals

Karen Koch MBChB FCDerm MMed
Clinical Specialist
Department of Dermatology
Wits Donald Gordon Medical Centre
Johannesburg, South Africa

Minal Patwardhan DVD MD
Medical Director and Specialist Dermatologist
Department of Dermatology
Minal Medical Centre
Dubai, UAE

Minu L Mathew MD
Junior Resident
Department of Dermatology
KVG Medical College and Hospital
Sullia, Karnataka, India

Ncoza C Dlova MBChB FCDerm PhD
Professor of Dermatology and Chief Specialist
Division of Dermatology
Nelson R Mandela School of Medicine
Durban, South Africa

Neha Meena MD
Specialist
Department of Dermatology
Central Hospital, NWR
Jaipur, Rajasthan, India

Safia Bashir MD
Senior Resident
Department of Dermatology, Venereology, and Leprology
Government Medical College
Srinagar, Jammu and Kashmir, India

Shilpa Garg DNB (Dermatology and Venereology)
Consultant Dermatologist
Department of Dermatology
Sir Ganga Ram Hospital
New Delhi, India

Sidharth Tandon MD
Senior Resident
Department of Dermatology
Dr Ram Manohar Lohia Hospital and Post Graduate Institute of Medical Education Research
New Delhi, India

Soumya Jagadeesan MD
Associate Professor
Department of Dermatology
Amrita Institute of Medical Sciences
Kochi, Kerala, India

Trilokraj Tejasvi MD
Assistant Professor
Department of Dermatology
University of Michigan
Ann Arbor, Michigan, USA

Yasmeen J Bhat MD FACP
Assistant Professor
Department of Dermatology
Venereology and Leprology
Government Medical College
Srinagar, Jammu and Kashmir, India

PREFACE

The subject of "sensitive skin" has always been intriguing, more so as very little literature exists on this. In practice, skin which is unable to tolerate repeated use of topical products, cosmetics, and cosmeceuticals is in essence "sensitive skin." This can refer to dry skin, red skin, easily irritated skin, and skin at different stages of life—in infancy, geriatric age, and even topical steroid damaged face. We, the editors, have tried to put together different aspects regarding care, treatment, and cosmetics on sensitive skin, if at all they need modifications. We have brought together global and Indian experts for this. We confess there is really very little literature on this; but that makes the venture even more exciting! Experts from all over the world have written on managing sensitive skin in different disease setups—acne, rosacea, and eczema among others. Special emphasis is also given to use of cosmetic products and dermatosurgical procedures in sensitive skin. The book is the need of the hour.

We hope you enjoy reading it as much as we enjoyed writing and editing it. We would like to thank our families (Srikanta Basu and Abhik Basu, Rashmi's family and Tarun Bhatnagar and Rishit, Surabhi's family) for bearing with us for the loss of time.

Rashmi Sarkar
Surabhi Sinha

CONTENTS

1. **What is Sensitive Skin?**   1
   Surabhi Sinha, Rashmi Sarkar

2. **Sensitive Skin Care: General Measures—Do's and Don'ts**   14
   Neha Meena, Surabhi Sinha, Rashmi Sarkar

3. **Skin Care of Acne Vulgaris in Sensitive Skin**   19
   Divya Arora, Shilpa Garg

4. **Skin Care in Sensitive Skin of Rosacea**   31
   Karen Koch, Ncoza C Dlova

5. **Topical Steroid Damaged/Dependent Face**   39
   Yasmeen J Bhat, Safia Bashir

6. **Skin Care in Dermatitis and Psoriasis in Patients with Sensitive Skin**   49
   Ambika Damodaran, Trilokraj Tejasvi

7. **Cosmetic Intolerance Syndrome**   57
   Surabhi Sinha

8. **Dermatological Products for Sensitive Skin: Practice Tips**   61
   Surabhi Sinha, Sidharth Tandon

9. **Care of Sensitive Skin in Newborns**   69
   Indrashis Podder, Rashmi Sarkar

10. **Skin Care of Aged Skin**   78
    Indrashis Podder, Rashmi Sarkar

11. **Cosmetics for Sensitive Skin: Practical Tips**   82
    Minal Patwardhan, Akreti S Sobti

12. **Dermatological Procedures in Sensitive Skin**   89
    Azin Ayatollahi, Alireza Firooz

The Sensitive Skin: Treatment Modalities and Cosmeceuticals

13. **Skin Care Products for Sensitive Skin: Soaps, Cleansers, and Shampoos** 97
    Soumya Jagadeesan, Minu L Mathew

14. **Moisturizers in Sensitive Skin** 104
    Surabhi Sinha

Index *113*

CHAPTER 1

What is Sensitive Skin?

Surabhi Sinha, Rashmi Sarkar

INTRODUCTION

Sensitive skin (SS) is described as a clinical phenomenon of hyperreactivity of the human skin, triggered by contact agents and/or mechanical and/or environmental factors, with varied symptoms, most frequently stinging, burning, itching, tightness, and smarting.[1,2] The symptoms may occur minutes to hours after a single contact or after several exposures to the agent, acting cumulatively.[3] Generally, substances considered innocuous or nonirritating for the general population are involved in the triggering of the symptoms.

The presence of symptoms in the absence of signs makes this entity a diagnostic challenge. No objective screening or diagnostic tests are currently available for routine clinic or hospital use. Thus it is mostly a clinically diagnosed condition and many "patients" self-diagnose themselves to have sensitive skin. Certain individuals may view sensitive skin as "fashionable," but sufferers and treating dermatologists both would agree that it is a bothersome condition to have or treat. It is a widely prevalent condition, with 52% of women reporting self-declared SS in a telephonic survey in the United States, while in the United Kingdom, a mail-based survey found SS in 51.5% women and 38.2% men.[4,5]

Even in the absence of a universally agreed-upon definition, a tenuous consensus in the literature is that sensitive skin is characterized by predominantly subjective symptoms without predictable classical visible signs of irritation and without an immunologic response.[6,7] Although transient redness, dryness, or tenderness may accompany adverse sensations, and sensitive skin may be less supple or hydrated, subjects often experience sensory effects only.[7,8] Subjective irritation, invisible irritation, nonimmunologic adverse skin reactions, nonimmunologic inflammation, and self-estimated enhanced skin sensitivity have been proposed as more clinically meaningful terms.[8-11] It is more likely to be an umbrella term encompassing distinct entities with various levels of sensitivities.

Due to the lack of easily discernible signs or proper diagnostic procedures, the entity has not found its due place in most dermatology textbooks. However, the interest in the condition is not merely limited to researchers. Before manufacturers introduce any new dermatological product into the market, both skin safety testing and risk assessment are performed to ensure skin compatibility.[12] Consumer sensitivity is commercially critical as well because it strongly influences consumer choice.[13] In fact, Jourdain et al. reported that nearly 78% of consumers with self-declared sensitive skin avoided certain products because of unpleasant sensory effects associated with their use.[14]

CLASSIFICATION SYSTEMS FOR SENSITIVE SKIN

Sensitive skin has been classified by different authors into different categories based on different parameters. Pons-Guiraud classified SS on the basis of inciting triggers into very sensitive (very dry, reacts to both exogenous and endogenous factors, strong psychological component), environmentally sensitive (dry, thin skin, blushes and flushes, reacts primarily to environmental factors), and cosmetically sensitive (transient reactivity to usually definable cosmetic agents).[6]

Muizzuddin on the other hand classified them on the basis of the primary pathology into delicate skin (easily disrupted barrier function), reactive skin (strong inflammatory response) and stingers (heightened neurosensory perception to minor stimulants).[15]

Baumann formulated the Baumann skin type indicator on the basis four dichotomous parameters to characterize facial skin types: dry or oily, sensitive or resistant, pigmented or nonpigmented, and wrinkled or unwrinkled.[16]

Sensitive skin can also be encountered in partially treated disorders with skin inflammation such as contact dermatitis, atopic dermatitis, seborrheic dermatitis, psoriasis, or rosacea. In such conditions, rarely, visible erythema with/without scaling may be seen. Thus, sensitive skin can be divided into visible and invisible types.

Visible Sensitive Skin

This refers to patients with evidence or known history of atopic dermatitis or eczema (including seborrheic dermatitis and contact dermatitis)/rosacea, each of them a prototype of the three postulated mechanisms of sensitive skin—barrier disruption, immune hyper-reactivity, and heightened neurosensory perception, respectively. Figure 1 shows a lady with contact dermatitis on the face with visible sensitive skin. Figure 2 shows a young girl with visible sensitive skin secondary to rosacea. Even these dermatoses may at times present atypically and be difficult to diagnose. Also their skin may not be functionally intact even when the dermatitis is apparently in remission, and they may develop sensitivity to innocuous typical agents.

Invisible Sensitive Skin

This is the more challenging group of patient with no obvious signs of inflammation at the time of contact with the dermatologist.

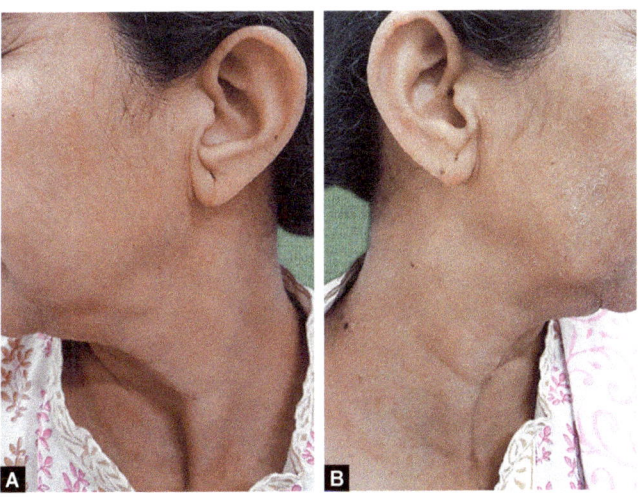

FIG.1: Clinical photograph showing erythema, dryness, and scaling in a patient with "visible" sensitive skin. *(For color version, see Plate 1)*

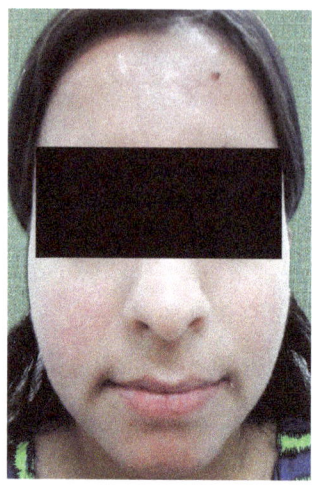

FIG. 2: Clinical photograph of a young patient of rosacea with sensitive skin. *(For color version, see Plate 1)*

A thorough search for any predisposing dermatosis, especially contact dermatitis, should be made and history and examination should be performed at each visit so as not to miss any clues to the antecedent cause. Many patients may simply have xerosis due to skin care products themselves, or diabetic thin dry skin. This group also includes patients who develop contact urticaria on contact with dermatological products and otherwise have quiescent skin.

FACTORS AFFECTING SENSITIVE SKIN[17]

Host Factors

Ethnicity

Skin types I-II have been believed to develop erythema more commonly than others.[18] Two large epidemiological studies have, however, disproved this difference.[14,19] Blacks are believed to be less reactive and Asians more reactive than Caucasians; but these data rarely reach statistical significance.[20]

Age

Young patients have been shown to have sensitive skin more commonly. Elderly patients have thin skin/impaired barriers so would be expected to have more sensitivity, but decreased tactile sensitivity decreases with age and so does the sensitivity.[1,2,21]

Sex

The condition was initially described in females and believed to be more common in females due to their thinner skin and hormonal factors, and greater exposure to cosmetic skin products. In fact, the majority of women surveyed in United States, Europe, and Japan believe that they have SS.[22] However, with changing times and greater use of both cosmetics and toiletries, and different fabrics by males as well, the rates of SS have increased in men too.[23] An almost equal incidence in both sexes is now believed to occur and was concluded by Farage in 2009 and later by Taieb et al. in their respective studies.[23,24]

Farage also found differences in the reasons to which both the sexes attributed their SS. Women sited dermatological and cosmetic products more commonly (18% vs. 11%) and men reported rubbing/friction from contact/fabrics more frequently (9% vs. 4%).[25]

Site of Body

Face is involved most commonly due to thin skin, more nerve endings, and greater cosmetics use. Farage reported SS in 77.3% individuals on the face, 60.7% on body and 56.3% on genital skin in a study on 1,039 men and women.[23] Sanit-Martory et al. also concluded face was the most common site flowed by hands, scalp, feet, neck, torso, and back.[26] On the face, Nasolabial fold is the most sensitive, followed by malar eminences, chin, forehead, and the upper lip in that order.[26,27] The genital skin is also of particular interest as it is derived from the embryonic endoderm and is the different from skin elsewhere.[28] Nonkeratinized vulvar skin clearly exhibits increased permeability and is thus, prone to sensitivity to topical hygiene products and topical medications, especially in case of overuse.[29]

Other Dermatoses

Atopic dermatitis (considered one of the causative factors now), seborrheic dermatitis, acne, rosacea, psoriasis, and contact dermatitis all lead to altered skin barrier or heightened neurosensory reactivity.[30] These are causes of "visible" sensitive skin, even when these diseases are in partial or total remission, the skin may look normal with minimal erythema or scaling, but the sensitivity may still be heightened.

Occupation

Cosmetics are considered the main triggers in a large proportion of patients. Occupations with greater cosmetic use may develop sensitive skins more frequently.

Environmental Factors

Low temperatures, humidity, wind, sun, and pollution all favor sensitivity of skin. Air conditioning is known to trigger symptoms of sensitive skin, thus leading to higher figures in summer than winters.

Fabrics and Sensitive Skin

Fabrics deserve a special mention due to their ubiquitous presence. A fraction of individuals with SS report intolerance to fabrics like clothes and towels. Softened (with liquid fabric conditioners) fabrics may be expected to be beneficial to them, even though studies of the effect of unsoftened fabrics on SS have revealed no adverse effects.[31-33]

Pierard et al. evaluated softened and unsoftened fabrics on normal and irritated (induced by sodium lauryl sulfate application) skin on 15 volunteers with SS.[33] Visual grading (redness, dryness, and smoothness), skin stripping, squamometry, and biophysical parameters measurement [capacitance, transepidermal water loss (TEWL), colorimetry] were performed. No adverse effects were seen with either of the fabrics but a mild beneficial effect was seen with the softened fabrics, especially on previously irritated skin. The volunteers themselves also favored the softened fabrics. The authors postulated that reduced mechanical friction by the softened fabrics (as the fibers were lubricated by the conditioner) was responsible for reduced disruption of corneocytes and hence reduces feeling of irritation.

TRIGGERS FOR SENSITIVE SKIN[6]

Table 1 highlights the various chemical, mechanical, and environment triggers for SS. Sensitivity to one or more triggers does not imply or predict sensitivity to others.[10]

Table 1: Triggers for sensitive skin

Chemical	Mechanical	Environmental
• Cosmetics • Toiletries • Sunscreens • Chemical exfoliants • Topical medications (especially topical steroids) • Household cleaning agents • Soaps and detergents • Water • Air pollutants • Endogenous hormones and stress-induced changes	• Fabrics • Sweating and maceration • Dermabrasion • Laser resurfacing • Facelift procedures • Local minor trauma	• Ultraviolet light • Heat • Cold • Windy conditions • Air conditioning • Humidity

PATHOGENESIS

It is not clearly understood why some patients develop sensitive skin. There is a decreased "tolerance threshold" of the skin, either due to: (i) heightened neurosensory response; and/or (ii) impaired skin barrier; and/or (iii) enhanced immune responsiveness. Though the pathogenesis is not completely elucidated yet, it strongly believed to NOT originate from the immune system.[24] Muizzuddin et al. studied these three parameters with objective biophysical measurements. Barrier function was tested with cellophane tape stripping of the stratum corneum (SC) followed by TEWL measurement. Altered immune reactivity was tested by onset and intensity of skin reaction to Balsam of Peru and sensorineural change was tested by the lactic acid stinging test.[15]

Seidnari et al. also evaluated biophysical parameters in patients with SS.[8] They assessed baseline biophysical parameters in SS patients, including TEWL, capacitance, pH, sebum, and skin color, and compared these with normal skin. They showed higher scores on the stinging test and the SS patients. Higher TEWL, higher pH, and higher colorimetric a* (red-green coordinate) values and lowered capacitance, lower sebum values and L* (lightness) values were seen in SS patients. However, only capacitance and a* values achieved statistical significance. They, thus concluded that skin barrier impairment and vascular hyper-reactivity are likely pathogenic factors in SS.

Histopathologically vasodilatation and inflammatory infiltrate are infrequent findings. Predisposing host factors in an individual with heightened neurosensory reactivity and/or impaired skin barrier (which could increase exposure to environmental irritants) along with environmental triggers is believed to cause sensitive skin.

Role of Impaired Skin Barrier

This is believed to be a key factor in the pathogenesis. Some author now consider atopic predisposition to be an independent predictive factor for SS. Cho et al. studied the difference in the quantity of SC ceramides on the face in individuals with sensitive skin and normal skin.[34] They performed extraction and high performance liquid chromatograph electrospray ionization mass spectrometry of the ceramides. They found that the mean value was significantly lower in the individuals with SS on the face. The SC ceramides are an integral constituent of the SC barrier and hence have an important role to play.

Role of Sensorineural Change

The prototype of this mechanism is patients of rosacea who even on remission of the rosacea symptoms continue to have sensitive skin. Recent literature has demonstrated a thermal receptor of transient potential vanilloid 1 (TRPV1) that can act as a facilitator of neurogenic inflammation.[35] TRPV1 is stimulated by chemicals, heat, cold, and capsaicin and is involved in causation of SS.[36,37]

Altered Immune Reactivity

This explains why patients of contact allergic dermatitis may continue to complain of sensitivity of the skin even after apparent resolution of the dermatitis.

CLINICAL FEATURES

Subjective sensory symptoms on an apparently normal looking skin is what basically constitutes sensitive skin. Though there are no clear signs, these patients may exhibit skins that are less

What is Sensitive Skin?

hydrated, less supple-looking, and more erythematous and more telangiectatic. The various symptoms described by patients include stinging, itching, tingling, prickling, and burning. These terms have been described by various authors to aid better understanding and description of symptoms by both patients and treating physicians.
- Stinging: A sensation that occurs when alcohol is applied to a cut on the skin/a sharp sensation like a pinprick or insect bite[38,39]
- Itching: Desire to scratch[38]
- Tingling: A lively "pins and needles" sensation[38]
- Prickling: Sensation caused by the movement of rough fabrics over skin[40]
- Burning: Painful sensation produced by extremes of temperature or chemical irritants.[38]

DIAGNOSIS OF SENSITIVE SKIN

Due to the absence of objective signs, self-assessment questionnaires are valid and logical tools. Jourdain et al. have given such questionnaires using assess facial skin neurosenstivity to capsaicin as a measure of the sensitivity of the skin.[41] No laboratory methods are in routine use currently and are mostly employed for research purposes only. Some authors have argued that the objective assessment of SS may not be possible and/or viable at all.[41] They found no statistically significant difference between the visual (erythema), and biophysical characteristics (TEWL, SC hydration, and blood perfusion) between SS and normal skin. This is in contrast to the work of other authors who have conducted objective studies and found differences between SS and normal skin.[8,15] Sensory reactivity to application of 10% lactic acid (LA) or capsaicin in nasolabial sulcus and saline solution in the other sulcus has been used most frequently and stinging evaluated. The LA stinging test is accepted and used widely but it lacks objectivity. Other tests include burning and erythema on sodium lauryl sulfate application, identification of tumor necrosis factors-alpha (TNF-α) and mast cell mediators in SS foci, magnetic resonance imaging of brain, epidermal function tests including TEWL measurement, and contact testing.[42]

Assessment of "subclinical irritation" may prove to be the breakthrough in evaluation of SS.[43] New noninvasive tests can detect subclinical damage and correlate well with the sensory perception too. Cross-polarized light is one such modality which can be used to detect subclinical irritation and predict sensitivity to possible irritants.

MANAGEMENT

"Two-week strategy" described by Draelos is followed:[3]
- Discontinue all cosmetics, topical dermatologic products, and over-the-counter products for 2 weeks at least
- Discontinue all topical medication for 2 weeks
- Eliminate source of skin irritation and prickle by selecting soft loose clothes
- Reevaluate after 2 weeks—check for any newly visible signs of visible SS—atopic dermatitis, contact dermatitis, rosacea, or acne. Treat them accordingly until 2 weeks after all visible signs of skin disease have disappeared
- Patch tests and photopatch tests to look for subclinical contact allergic/photocontact dermatitis in invisible SS
- Test for contact urticaria
- Facial sting testing with 10% lactic acid to one nasolabial fold and normal saline to the other fold
- Allow the female patient to add one facial cosmetic at a time in the following order: lipstick, face powder, and blush
- Moisturizers and optimized lipid mixes can improve impaired barrier function
- Avoid-water based moisturizers as they may cause dryness sooner and they contain more preservatives
- Cleansers used should be acidic or neutral pH as alkaline pH in harsh cleansers can derange the skin barrier more rapidly
- Anti-inflammatory (e.g., flavonoids), antioxidants (to scavenge the very strong irritants-free radicals), and vanilloid receptor antagonists also help in improvement2
- Use test cosmetics by applying them to a 2 cm area lateral to the eye for at least five consecutive nights. Cosmetics to be tested in the following order: mascara, eye-liner, eyebrow pencil, eye shadow, facial foundation, blush, facial powder, and any other colored facial cosmetic
- Make a list of ingredients/products that the patient ought to avoid.

Thus, it is a long-drawn and challenging process requiring patience on the part of both the patient and treating dermatologist.

REFERENCES

1. Farage MA, Katsarou A, Maibach HI. Sensitive skin. Sensory, clinical, and physiological factors. In: Borel AO, Paye M, Maibach HI, editors. Handbook of cosmetic science and technology. 4th ed. Boca Raton: CRC Press/Taylor & Francis Group; 2014. pp. 59-69.
2. Berardesca E, Farage M, Maibach H. Sensitive skin: An overview. Int J Cosmet Sci. 2013;35:2-8.
3. Draelos ZD. Sensitive skin: perceptions, evaluation, and treatment. Am J Contact Dermat. 1997;8:67-78.
4. Simion FA, Rau AH. Sensitive skin: What it is and how to formulate for it. Cosmet Toiletries. 1994;109:43-9.
5. Amin S, Maibach HI. Cosmetic intolerance syndrome: Pathophysiology and management. Cosmet Dermatol. 1996;9:34-42.
6. Pons-Guiraud A. Sensitive skin: A complex and multifactorial syndrome. J Cosmetic Dermatol. 2005;3:145-8.
7. Coverly J, Peters L, Whittle E, et al. Susceptibility to skin stinging, non-immunologic contact urticaria and acute skin irritation; is there a relationship? Contact Dermatitis. 1998;38:90-5.
8. Seidenari S, Francomano M, Mantovani L. Baseline biophysical parameters in subjects with sensitive skin. Contact Dermatitis. 1998;38:311-5.
9. Simion FA, Rhein LD, Morrison BM Jr, et al. Self-perceived sensory responses to soap and synthetic detergent bars correlate with clinical signs of irritation. J Am Acad Dermatol. 1995;32:205-11.
10. Marriott M, Holmes J, Peters L, et al. The complex problem of sensitive skin. Contact Dermatitis. 2005;53:93-9.
11. Loffler H, Dickel H, Kuss O, et al. Characteristics of self-estimated enhanced skin susceptibility. Acta Derm Venereol. 2001;81:343-6.
12. Robinson MK. Racial differences in acute and cumulative skin irritation responses between. Caucasian Asian Populations. 2000;42:134-43.
13. Reilly DM, Ferdinando D, Johnston C, et al. The epidermal nerve fibre network: Characterization of nerve fibres in human skin by confocal microscopy and assessment of racial variations. Br J Dermatol. 1997;137(2):163-70.
14. Jourdain R, De Lacharriere O, Bastien P, et al. Ethnic variations in self-perceived sensitive skin: epidemiological survey. Contact Dermatitis. 2002;45:162-69.
15. Muizzuddin N, Marenus KD, Maes DH. Factors defining sensitive skin and its treatment. Am J Contact Dermat. 1998;9:170-5.
16. Baumann L. Understanding and treating various skin types: the Baumann skin type indicator. Dermatol Clin. 2008;26:359-73.
17. Farage MA. Sensitive skin: Closing in on a physiological cause. Contact Dermatitis. 2010;62:137-49.

18. Lev-Tov H, Maibach HI. The sensitive skin syndrome. Indian J Dermatol. 2012;57: 419-23.
19. Willis CM, Shaw S, De Lacharriere O, et al. Sensitive skin: an epidemiological study. Br J Dermatol. 2001;145:258-63.
20. Modjtahed SP, Maibach HI. Ethnicity as a possible endogenous factor in irritant contact dermatitis: Comparing the irritant responses among Caucasian, Blacks and Asians. Contact Dermatitis. 2002;47:272-8.
21. Farage MA. Perceptions of sensitive skin with age. In: Farage MA, Miller KW, Maibach HI, editors. Textbook of aging skin. Berlin-Heidelberg: Springer-Verlag; 2010. pp. 1027-46.
22. Kligman A. Human models for characterizing "sensitive skin." Cosm Derm. 2001; 14:15-9.
23. Farage MA. How do perceptions of sensitive skin differ at different anatomical sites? An epidemiological study. Clin Exp Dermatol. 2009;38:e521-30.
24. Taieb C, Auges M, Georgescu V, et al. Sensitive skin in Brazil and Russia: An epidemiological and comparative approach. Eur J Dermatol. 2014;24:372-6.
25. Farage MA. Does sensitive skin differ between men and women? Cutan Ocul Toxicol. 2010;29:153-63.
26. Saint-Martory C, Roguedas-Contios AM, Sibaud V, et al. Sensitive skin is not limited to the face. Br J Dermatol. 2008;158:130-33.
27. Marriott M, Holmes J, Peters L, et al. The complex problem of sensitive skin. Contact Dermatitis. 2005;53:93-9.
28. Farage MA, Maibach HI. The vulvar epithelium differs from the skin: Implications for cutaneous testing to address topical vulvar exposures. Contact Dermatitis. 2004;51:201-9.
29. Tagami H. Racial differences on skin barrier function. Cutis. 2002;70:6-7; discussion 21-3.
30. Farage MA, Bowtell P, Katsarou A. Self-diagnosed sensitive skin in women with clinically diagnosed atopic dermatitis. Clin Med Dermatol. 2008;2:21-8.
31. Hatch KL. Chemicals and textiles I – Dermatological problems related to fiber content and dyes. Text Res J. 1984;54:664-82.
32. Hatch KL. Chemicals and textiles (II). Dermatological problems related to finishes. Text Res J. 1984;54:721-32.
33. Pierard GE, Arrese JE, Rodriguez C, et al. Effects of softened and unsoftened fabrics on sensitive skin. Contact Dermatitis. 1994;30:286-91.
34. Cho HJ, Chung Y, Lee HB, et al. Quantitative study of stratum corneum ceramides contents in patients with sensitive skin. J Dermatol. 2012;39:295-300.
35. Richters R, Falcone D, Uzunbajakava N, et al. What is Sensitive skin? A systematic literature review of objective measurements. Skin Pharmacol Physiol. 2015;28:75-83.
36. Aubdool AA, Brain SD. Neurovascular aspects of skin neurogenic inflammation. J Investig Dermatol Symp Proc. 2011;15:33-9.
37. Costa A, Eberlin S, Polettini AJ, et al. Neuromodulatory and anti-inflammatory ingredients for sensitive skin: in vitro assessment. Inflamm Allergy Drug Targets. 2014;13:191-8.

38. Green BG, Bluth J. Measuring the chemosensory irritability of human skin. J Toxicol Cutans Ocul Toxicol. 1995;14:23-48.
39. Green BG. Regional and individual differences in cutaneous sensitivity to chemical irritants: Capsaicin and menthol. J Toxicol Cutan Ocul Toxicol. 1996;15:277-95.
40. McMohan SB, Koltzenberg M. Itching for an explanation. Trends Neurosci. 1992;15:497-501.
41. Diogo L, Papoila AL. Is it possible to characterize objectively sensitive skin? Skin Res Technol. 2010;16:30-7.
42. Jourdain R, Bastien P, de Lacharriere O, et al. Detection thresholds of capsaicin: A new test to assess facial skin neurosenstivity. J Cosmet Sci. 2005;56:153-66.
43. Simion FA, Rhein LD, Morrison BM, et al. Self-perceived sensory responses to soap and synthetic detergent bars correlate with clinical signs of irritation. J Am Acad Dermatol. 1995;32:205-11.

CHAPTER 2

Sensitive Skin Care: General Measures—Do's and Don'ts

Neha Meena, Surabhi Sinha, Rashmi Sarkar

INTRODUCTION

Sensitive skin, also known as reactive/hyper-reactive/intolerant or irritable skin, is defined as the onset of erythema and/or prickling, burning, or tingling sensations due to various chemical, physical, and psychological factors.[1] Individuals with sensitive skin may have cutaneous barrier dysfunction with or without increased neurosensory input or high immune responsiveness.[1] Sensitive skin can be classified depending upon the clinical sensitivities and probable causative factors, according to either Pons-Guiraud classification or Muizzuddin classification.[1,2] Sensitive skin care ranges from identifying the cause and its avoidance and use of gentle cleansers, to repairing and restoring the cutaneous barrier by frequent use of moisturizers.[3,4]

GENERAL MEASURES—DO'S AND DON'TS FOR CARE OF SENSITIVE SKIN

- Discontinue all the topical skin products including soaps, prescription medications, and cosmetics at least for 2 weeks. This will help in diagnosis of underlying cutaneous diseases (if any) and thus, its treatment especially contact dermatitis. This will also reduce the symptoms of sensitive skin. In severe cases, washout period up to 12 months may be needed.[1,5] At the most, a mild soap or cleanser could be used sparingly
- Cosmetic products use should be minimal and only if necessary
- Use specially formulated bland products for sensitive skin with one or very few ingredients

Sensitive Skin Care: General Measures—Do's and Don'ts

- Use syndet (synthetic detergent) bars
- Use nonrinsing cleansing lotions or thermal spring water spritzers. Use tissue paper to gentle patting. Avoid toweling or rubbing the face
- Fragrance free products with pure ingredients should be used[6]
- Fresh cosmetics with usually less than 10 ingredients, low-allergenic potential, easily removable with water should be used[1]
- Powder cosmetics are preferred as they may contain non allergen and nonirritants agents such as titanium dioxide, talc, aluminum oxide, and silicates, e.g., powder facial foundation.[5] Use black-colored eyeliner, eyebrow pencils and mascara with light earth tone eye shadows[1]
- Physical sunscreens should be preferred
- Avoidance of nail polishes
- Chemicals such as alcohol, propylene glycol, butylene glycol, cocamidopropyl betaine, and triethanolamine are common irritants in cosmetics and shampoos. So, these should be avoided[7]
- Avoid chemical peelings with exfoliants as trichloroacetic acid, α-hydroxy acids, retinol, resorcinol, or salicylic acid. Depending on the concentration and on the pH in the final formulation, they can be very irritating and an aggravating factor for sensitive skin.[7,8] Very mild peels like lactic acid peels are preferred
- Choose moisturizing creams with a bland texture and one or two ingredients only
- Due care of skin should be taken to avoid excess sun exposure, temperature variation, and wind chapping
- Reapply as and when required, especially in case of exposure to air conditioning or overly heated environment.[2,7] A humidified atmosphere may help
- Moisturizers also help in restoration of softness and suppleness of the skin, improve skin homeostasis, and relieve the dryness[9]
- Patients of rosacea mostly have sensitive skin. Cosmetics and toiletries containing alcohol, menthol, peppermint, eucalyptus, and clove oils can exacerbate rosacea. So, their skin products should not contain the known irritants and allergens.[3] Use of gentle cleanser followed by moisturizer can help in repair and maintaining the stratum corneum-barrier function, increased cutaneous hydration, and lower the chances of the sensitive skin syndrome[10]

- Use hair products without irritating tension-active surfactants
- Avoid hair products with ammonia and formaldehyde
- Discontinue the use of product which causes burning and discomfort
- Avoid hot and spicy food and caffeine, if skin becomes more irritable after their consumption
- Prolonged use of topical corticosteroids should be avoided as they lead to increase skin fragility and lead to telangiectases, chronic persistent, and localized erythema. This may further result into increased cosmetic intolerance and sensitive skin[5]
- Products containing 4-t-butylcyclohexanol and acetyl dipeptide-1 cetyl ester can be used to alleviate sensory effects in sensitive skin. These compounds counteract the hyper-responsiveness of nerve fibers by their[11]
- Anti-inflammatory agent licochalcone A can also be used in cosmetic products for sensitive skin
- Crisaborole (2%) topical ointment is a nonsteroidal, anti-inflammatory, phosphodiesterase-4 inhibitor that can be used in sensitive skin, especially in sensitive skins, atopic dermatitis, and psoriasis[12]
- Dermatological procedures/therapies such as phototherapy, chemical peeling, derma roller, dermabrasion, laser resurfacing, and facelifts can all aggravate skin sensitivity. Postoperative skin care should be taken[2]
- Anti-aging creams with sodium salicylate should be preferred over those containing salicylic acid. Higher concentration of salicylic acid in anti-aging products can cause adverse effects such as somatosensory and visible irritation[13]
- Hydroxy acids in anti-aging cream should be replaced by polyhydroxy and bionic acids, as they are nonirritant, also acts as antioxidant, moisturizer, and repair skin barrier[14]
- Use of moisturizers containing squalene and 5% colloidal oatmeal helps in reducing and preventing the symptoms of sensitive skin[15-17]
- Maintenance of cutaneous pH (5.5 on the surface) keeps the whole barrier and adequate hydration of the skin[18]
- Use of synthetic pseudoceramide can also help in compensating natural ceramide and restoration of skin barrier function[19,20]

- One should look for depression and neuropsychiatric signs if sensitive skin symptoms persist even after the proper care and protection
- Body dysmorphic disorder should always be considered as differential while evaluating sensitive skin syndrome, especially when there are skin complaints without any objective findings counseling to be done to prevent recurrence.[2,7]

CONCLUSION

Sensitive skin care includes identification and avoidance of causative agent. Syndet bars, nonrinsing cleansing lotions, specially formulated fragrance free products with fewer ingredients, or products containing 4-t-butylcyclohexanol, acetyl dipeptide-1 cetyl, licochalcone A or crisaborole (2%) can be used to alleviate the symptoms of sensitive skin. Moisturisers containing squalene, 5% colloidal oatmeal or synthetic pseudo-ceramide should be preferred for epidermal repair in sensitive skin.

REFERENCES

1. Inamadar AC, Palit A. Sensitive skin: An overview. Indian J Dermatol Venereol Leprol. 2013;79(1):9-16.
2. Pons-Guiraud A. Sensitive skin: A complex and multifactorial syndrome. J Cosmet Dermatol. 2004;3(3):145-8.
3. Grivet-Seyve M, Santoro F, Lachmann N. Evaluation of a novel very high sun-protection-factor moisturizer in adults with rosacea-prone sensitive skin. Clin Cosmet Investig Dermatol. 2017;10:211-9.
4. Misery L, Stander S, Szepietowski JC, et al. Definition of sensitive skin: An expert position paper from the special interest group on sensitive skin of the International Forum for the Study of Itch. Acta Derm Venereol. 2017;97(1):4-6.
5. Fisher AA. "Status cosmeticus": a cosmetic intolerance syndrome. Cutis. 1990;46(2):109-10.
6. Lev-Tov H, Maibach HI. The sensitive skin syndrome. Indian J Dermatol. 2012;57(6):419-23.
7. Escalas-Taberner J, Gonzalez-Guerra E, Guerra-Tapia A. Sensitive skin: A complex syndrome. Actas Dermo-Sifiliograficas. 2011;102(8):563-71.
8. Ehnis-Perez A, Torres-Alvarez B, Cortes-Garcia D, et al. Relationship between transient receptor potential vanilloid-1 expression and the intensity of sensitive skin symptoms. J Cosmet Dermatol. 2016;15(3):231-7.
9. Draelos ZD, Ertel K, Berge C. Niacinamide-containing facial moisturizer improves skin barrier and benefits subjects with rosacea. Cutis. 2005;76(2):135-41.

10. Del Rosso JQ, Thiboutot D, Gallo R, et al. Consensus recommendations from the American Acne & Rosacea Society on the management of rosacea, part 1: a status report on the disease state, general measures, and adjunctive skin care. Cutis. 2013;92(5):234-40.
11. Schoelermann AM, Jung KA, Buck B, et al. Comparison of skin calming effects of cosmetic products containing 4-t-butylcyclohexanol or acetyl dipeptide-1 cetyl ester on capsaicin-induced facial stinging in volunteers with sensitive skin. J Eur Acad Dermatol Venereol. 2016;30(Suppl 1):18-20.
12. Zane LT, Hughes MH, Shakib S. Tolerability of crisaborole ointment for application on sensitive skin areas: A randomized, double-blind, vehicle-controlled study in healthy volunteers. Am J Clin Dermatol. 2016;17(5):519-26.
13. Merinville E, Byrne AJ, Rawlings AV, et al. Three clinical studies showing the anti-aging benefits of sodium salicylate in human skin. J Cosmet Dermatol. 2010;9(3):174-84.
14. Green BA, Yu RJ, Van Scott EJ. Clinical and cosmeceutical uses of hydroxyacids. Clin Dermatol. 2009;27(5):495-501.
15. Matheson JD, Clayton J, Muller MJ. The reduction of itch during burn wound healing. J Burn Care Rehab. 2001;22(1):76-81.
16. Sethi A, Kaur T, Malhotra SK, et al. Moisturizers: The slippery road. Indian J Dermatol. 2016;61(3):279-87.
17. Pazyar N, Yaghoobi R, Kazerouni A, et al. Oatmeal in dermatology: A brief review. Indian J Dermatol Venereol Leprol. 2012;78(2):142-5.
18. Duarte I, Silveira J, Hafner MF, et al. Sensitive skin: review of an ascending concept. An Bras Dermatol. 2017;92(4):521-5.
19. Isoda K, Nakamura T, Yoshida K, et al. The efficacy of a lip balm containing pseudo-ceramide on the dry lips of sensitive skin-conscious subjects. J Cosmet Dermatol. 2018;17(1):84-9.
20. Imokawa G. Role of ceramide in the barrier function of the stratum corneum, implications for the pathogenesis of atopic dermatitis. J Clin Exper Dermatol Res. 2014;05(01).

Skin Care of Acne Vulgaris in Sensitive Skin

Divya Arora, Shilpa Garg

INTRODUCTION

Acne vulgaris is a common disorder with which patient presents to dermatology outpatient department.[1] It is a disease of adolescent age group, majority of the patients present around puberty and it affects nearly 85% of teenagers.[2] However, we do see patients across all ages, in neonates, post adolescence (adult onset acne), and old age (senile acne). Acne affects 9.4% of the global population. In view of this high prevalence rate, it was once believed to be physiological but it is now defined as a chronic inflammatory disease of the pilosebaceous unit.[3]

The pathogenesis of acne is multifactorial with primarily the following etiological factors:
- Increased activity of sebaceous glands leading to seborrhoea
- Increased keratinization with abnormal follicular differentiation
- Microbial over activity with a secondary inflammatory response
- Role of androgens
- Presence of proinflammatory lipids.

Along with this, genetics, neuroendocrine regulatory mechanisms, diet, and other exogenous factors play an important role in the causation of acne.[3]

Their onset in adolescence and the associated psychosocial and emotional issues at that age affect the self-confidence and self-image of the patient. The course of acne is usually prolonged and they heal with sequelae like postinflammatory hyperpigmentation and scarring. These persist long after the active lesions have disappeared

and contribute to the persistent anxiety and stress.[4,5] It is because of the psychosocial issues that a patient seeks treatment. In a case of acne vulgaris, detailed history and examination are essential to check for the patient's skin type. Some of them have good tolerability, whereas some have a very sensitive skin. Among patients who have a sensitive skin, there may be two categories:
1. Patient with an inherently sensitive skin
2. Patients with secondary skin sensitivity due to multitude of topical applications.

INHERENTLY SENSITIVE SKIN

Sensitive skin has been defined clinically,[6-9] as the occurrence of abnormal stinging, burning, pain, pruritus, and tingling sensations in response to multiple factors. As discussed earlier, multiple classification systems have been proposed in an attempt to describe the types of sensitive skin. Yokota et al. defined three different types based on physiological parameters:[10]

- Type 1: Defined as a low barrier function group with high trans-epidermal water loss (TEWL) and abnormal desquamation
- Type 2: Defined as an inflammation group with normal barrier function and inflammatory changes
- Type 3: Defined as a neurosensitive group in terms of normal barrier function and no inflammatory changes.

ROLE OF SENSITIVE SKIN IN PATHOGENESIS OF ACNE

Development of acne is related in some aspects to the presence of sensitive skin. There are studies that show the presence of markers of subclinical inflammation in an acne prone skin even before the presence of follicular hyperkeratinization. It is both the surface epidermis and the follicular epithelium which contribute to the barrier function of skin.[11]

Baumann classified sensitive skin based on diagnosis (Box 1).[12] This classification throws more light on the relationship between sensitive skin and acne. According to him, the S1 sensitive skin is characterized by acne breakouts which may be in the form of comedones, papules, or pustules. He has assigned acne and acne prone skin to an altogether independent class of sensitive skin.

BOX 1	Baumann sensitive skin classification
Type 1: Pimples and comedones	
Type 2: Flushing	
Type 3: Burning and stinging or itching	
Type 4: Impaired barrier, contact, and irritant	

Surface Epithelium

In a study by Yamamoto et al., there was an increased TEWL, reduced stratum corneum hydration, and reduced intercellular lipid membrane components, namely, sphingosine and ceramides on the surface epidermis in patients with acne compared to healthy adults.[13] Emphasis is now being laid on the presence of inherent barrier abnormalities in acne patients so that specific management can be offered.[13]

Follicular Epithelium

The epithelium lining the sebaceous ducts is also responsible for maintaining barrier function of skin. Fillagrin is an important protein involved in the process of epidermal differentiation and helps in maintaining its integrity. It has been observed that the levels of fillagrin in the follicular epithelium were higher in acne lesions. Also, the inflammation incited by *Propionibacterium acnes* can further damage the perifollicular barrier. It is known to stimulate fillagrin expression in cultured keratinocytes.[14-17] Further studies are required to confirm if skin barrier changes precede acne or occur secondary to their pathogenesis.

SECONDARY SKIN SENSITIVITY DUE TO MULTITUDE OF TOPICAL APPLICATIONS

In an attempt to get past all the physical and psychological issues associated with acne, majority of patients use home remedies, medicate themselves, subject the skin to a number of known and unknown chemicals, and try different therapies in parlor and expose their skin to a multitude of physical and chemical agents before they actually reach a dermatologist. They are patients with high stress levels, low patience, poor tolerability and type 1 and 2 sensitive skin types.

The Sensitive Skin: Treatment Modalities and Cosmeceuticals

Keeping in view the above mentioned pathogenesis, the incidence of acne in patients with sensitive skin is high and the fact that some patients might be sensitized to common medicaments, the care of patient needs to be modified accordingly at every level (Box 2). Careful selection of products when dealing with a patient of acne with sensitive skin is essential to avoid the otherwise vicious cycle which ensues when both the conditions are treated as two separate entities (Fig. 1).

BOX 2	Levels of intervention

- Antiacne medications
    - Topical
    - Systemic
- Management of postinflammatory pigmentation
- Management of acne scars
    - Preprocedure
    - During procedure
    - Postprocedure care
- Routine skin care, cleansing and moisturizing
- Diet and lifestyle management

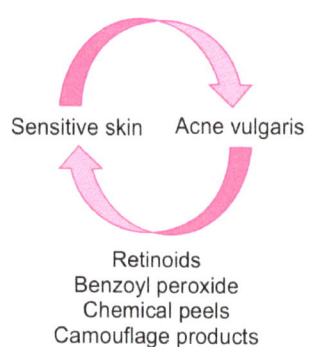

FIG. 1: Attempts at soothing a sensitive skin might aggravate acne and medications used to treat acne may worsen a sensitive skin leading to a vicious cycle.

TOPICAL ANTIACNE MEDICATIONS
Benzoyl Peroxide
Benzoyl peroxide is a topical formulation that is prescribed in all grades of acne. It is an oxidizing agent which works as an anti-acne antibacterial agent. It has a major role in preventing the emergence of resistant bacterial strains. It is lipophilic, penetrates the pilosebaceous duct, and acts on both surface and ductal *Propionibacterium acnes*. Application of benzoyl peroxide, however, has shown to increase TEWL and cause lipid peroxidation. It also leads to oxidation of the stratum corneum antioxidants and hence impairs the permeability barrier. This manifests clinically as cutaneous irritation which might be subjective or sensory or in the form of erythema and scaling in some.[18] In patients with sensitive skin, this response is exaggerated and hence caution should be exercised while prescribing it. It is available in different strengths, namely, 2.5, 3.5, and 5% cream formulations. Lower concentrations are preferred in patients with poor tolerance. Also, hydrophase base or microsphere formulations are more acceptable with gradual release of this potentially irritating drug. These improve treatment outcomes and ensure more patient compliance.[19] Supplementation with topical vitamin E helps in reducing the markers of lipid peroxidation.[20] Also, short contact treatment should be used if and when benzoyl peroxide is prescribed to these patients.

Topical Retinoids
All transretinoic acid (tretinoin), retinoic acid, retinaldehyde, and adapalene are various topical formulations available for treatment of acne. Retinoids work by alterations in epidermal keratinization and differentiation, downregulation of toll-like receptor-2 expression, decrease in dermal matrix degradation that is promoted by chronic photo damage, and alteration of various transcription factors involved in patterns of cutaneous inflammation.[21] Though an extremely useful class of drug, most common adverse effects are dryness, skin irritation, and TEWL. These adverse effects in part are due to their mechanism of action on the epidermis and dermis itself. As topical retinoids enhance desquamation with a reduction in stratum corneum thickness and function, alteration in permeability barrier function is a likely consequence.[22] The effects are usually

transient but may be prolonged in patients with pre-existing sensitive skin. Thus, they may have to be prescribed in sensitive skins with utmost caution.

These can be prevented by initially starting the patient on a barrier repair moisturizing cream to soothe the already irritated skin. A number of times patients self-initiate their use.[23] Hence an appropriate product should be suggested right at the beginning of treatment followed by introduction of retinol preparation once in 3 days or alternate day and then gradually increasing the frequency of application every 3-4 weeks. Strength of retinol used is also gradually increased. By then the skin adapts and the medication is better tolerated till the initial "retinization period" passes off.

Newer preparations like microspheres or incorporation into complex polymers are techniques used to avoid the cutaneous adverse effects because of the controlled slow release. Use of gel preparations over cream may be helpful. Also, 0.1% adapalene, which is a third-generation retinoid, has a better risk/benefit ratio in acne patients as compared to others.[24]

Shedding of superficial layers of stratum corneum make the skin more sensitive to sun exposure. Sunscreen is an essential coprescription. A water based or noncomedogenic sunscreen is needed to prevent aggravation of the process of comedogenesis. However in patients with sensitive skin, it is best to use a mineral zinc oxide or titanium based sunscreen.

Tightness or excessive stretching of skin should be taken as an early sign of intolerance to retinoids and hence adequate moisture control is required.[25]

Topical Antibacterial

Antibiotic creams and lotions are usually less irritating than antibiotic gels or serums. Antiacne antibacterial creams normally do not pose a risk to sensitive skin. However their prolonged usage at times may alter the normal flora of the skin and lead to development of resistant strains or gram-negative folliculitis.[26]

Fixed-dose Formulations

Fixed-dose preparations of different antiacne medications are available and useful especially in patients who do not tolerate benzoyl peroxide and retinoids well. Combination of niacinamide with benzoyl peroxide reduces irritation caused by benzoyl peroxide. Similarly, combining a topical antibacterial with retinoid has reduced the incidence of retinoid dermatitis.

ORAL MEDICATIONS
Tetracyclines
Tetracyclines, namely, doxycycline and minocycline, are relatively safe medications except that they sensitize the skin to sunlight and patient needs regular sun protection. Sunscreens limit the free radical damage from ultraviolet rays and serve to protect the epidermal barrier and underlying skin. As discussed earlier, physical sunscreens are better suited for this purpose in an acne prone skin. Minocycline induced pigmentation of the inflamed skin would be more in a previously damaged skin as compared to otherwise so it should be used with caution.

Isotretinoin
One of the most effective medicine and drug of choice for grade 4 acne or truncal acne, oral isotretinoin, has revolutionized the way acne is treated. It increases epidermal turnover, reduces the number of desmosomes and tonofilaments, and the cohesiveness between cells of stratum corneum leading to desquamation. Therefore, before the onset of its comedolytic activity, patients experience dryness, flaking, and increased photosensitivity. It also has a sebo-suppressive effect leading to alteration in cutaneous microflora with increased risk of gram-positive bacterial colonization. A sensitive skin which is already prone to provocation by minimal stimuli reacts more strongly. Hence, extra care should be taken in such patients with very low or intermittent doses and gradual increments in isotretinoin dosage and coprescription with a barrier repair moisturizer containing soothing humectants and emollients.[27-30]

POSTINFLAMMATORY HYPERPIGMENTATION AND SCAR MANAGEMENT
It is mainly the grade 3 and grade 4 acne which leads to postinflammatory hyperpigmentation and scarring, respectively. Various

interventions may be required to take care of the residual effect. A variety of chemical peeling agents are available in the market. Alpha-hydroxy acids (AHAs) and beta-hydroxy acids (BHAs) are the commonly used ones. Before starting a patient on any of these, sufficient prepeel preparation should be done. Skin should be hydrated and moisturized well. Vigorous washing or rubbing with acetone is avoided in patients with sensitive skin. It strips off the upper layers of stratum corneum along with superficial lipids. This may lead to deeper penetration of the AHA or BHA applied thereafter. Post-peel, patient should be advised to use ceramide/natural moisturizing factor based moisturizer to ensure quick healing along with strict sun protection. Q-switched Nd:YAG (neodymium-doped yttrium aluminum garnet) and intense pulsed light can be used to treat pigmentation, pores and acne, and to a small degree, skin texture, During procedures like microdermabrasion and CO_2 laser for scar management, similar precautions should be followed for a smoother recovery.

Fractional ablative lasers should be preferred over conventional ablative lasers, namely, the fractional CO_2 and erbium:YAG lasers, as they work through inducing microthermal zones leaving healthy skin cells in between, therefore, promoting faster healing and recovery. The importance of sun protection and moisturizing cannot be emphasized more post procedure.

ROUTINE SKIN CARE

Cleansing

Acne prone skin as discussed earlier has some amount of inherent sensitivity, weak epidermal barrier, and is prone to dryness. Add to it the topical medications with xerosis and cutaneous irritation as a common side effect; skin in patients with acne needs to be cleansed gently to remove the oil and dirt, without disturbing the internal milieu. Thus, an ideal cleanser in acne prone skin should not only be noncomedogenic and hydrating, but also non allergenic. At the outset patient should be counseled against overzealous and frequent washing of face. This not only makes the skin dry and disrupts the epidermal barrier but also may lead to acne detergens.[31-34] Soap free cleansers with a pH similar to that of skin are preferred. They should be paraben, alcohol, and fragrance free. Cleansers with additional BHA should be avoided in patients with sensitive skin. There is a wide spectrum of skin cleansing agents for acne prone patients ranging from lipid free cleansers, syndets, astringents, exfoliants, and abrasives. Liquid facial cleansers are highly effective and beneficial for sensitive skin. These can also be used synergistically with topical or systemic therapy. A mild cleansing agent does not interfere with the process of healing post chemical peel or other invasive procedures.[34]

Moisturizing

Moisturizers form an important component of the anti-acne armamentarium as they not only help in maintaining a healthy skin barrier but also reduce the adverse effects that may arise from anti-acne medications. Moisturizers are primarily composed of occlusives, emollients, and/or humectants. In acne prone skin, a moisturizer with nongreasy, silicone-based occlusives like dimethicone or cyclomethicone is preferred. Dimethicone reduces TEWL without a greasy feel and contains both occlusive and emollient properties. It is suitable for acne in sensitive patients as it is noncomedogenic and hypoallergenic. Cyclomethicone is a thicker silicone that has similar properties as dimethicone.[35] Other ingredients including topical medications for acne and botanical anti-inflammatory substances are sometimes added to moisturizers for acne. Zinc is being used in moisturizers because of its anti-inflammatory properties. Alkaline phosphatase requires multiple zinc ions, which are involved in adenosine monophosphate metabolism. This action has a role in restraining an inflammatory response. Other anti-inflammatory agents that have been tried in large number of moisturizers include aloe vera extract (in concentration >10%) and witch hazel containing high tannin levels.

LIFESTYLE MANAGEMENT

Acne patients require a more holistic approach; it is prudent that apart from medications and drugs, an analysis of hormonal and dietary components be done in order to reduce the load of topical agents being used. Role of low glycemic diet should be emphasized.

Foods with a higher glycemic index increase the demand for insulin and contribute toward insulin resistance. They should be avoided and those rich in proteins such as poultry, fish, lean meat, wholegrain breads, pasta, and fruits are recommended.[36]

CONCLUSION

To provide optimal treatment outcomes for patients with acne vulgaris with components of skin sensitivity, a thorough dedicated patient evaluation, careful selection of pharmacological interventions, and inclusion of an adjunctive skin care regime avoids skin tolerability reactions. Topical, systemic, and adjuvant treatments should be individualized after examining the patient as a whole to deliver best results.

REFERENCES

1. Tan JK, Bhate K. A global perspective on the epidemiology of acne. Br J Dermatol. 2015;172 (Suppl 1):3-12.
2. James WD. Acne. N Engl J Med. 2005;352:1463-72.
3. Layton AM, Eady EA, Zouboulis CC. Acne. In: Griffiths C, Barker J, Bleiker T, editors. Rook's textbook of dermatology. UK: Blackwell Publishing; 2016. p. 90.1.
4. Hazarika N, Archana M. The psychosocial impact of acne vulgaris. Indian J Dermatol. 2016;61(5):515-20.
5. Del Rosso JQ, Gold M, Rueda MJ, et al. Efficacy, safety, and subject satisfaction of a specified skin care regimen to cleanse, medicate, moisturize, and protect the skin of patients under treatment for acne vulgaris. J Clin Aesthet Dermatol. 2015;8:22-30.
6. Berardesca E, Fluhr JW, Maibach HI. What is sensitive skin? In: Berardesca E, Fluhr JW, Maibach HI, editors. Dermatology: Clinical and basic science series, sensitive skin syndrome. New York: Taylor and Francis Group; 2006. pp. 1-5.
7. Misery L. How the skin reacts to environmental factors. J Eur Acad Dermatol Venereol. 2007;21(2):5-8.
8. Farage MA, Maibach HI. Sensitive skin: New findings yield new insights. In: Textbook of cosmetic dermatology. Baran R, Maibach HI, editors. London: Informa Healthcare; 2010. p. 558.
9. Slodownik D, Williams J, Lee A, et al. Controversies regarding the sensitive skin syndrome. Expert Rev Dermatol. 2007;2:579-84.
10. Yokota T, Matsumoto M, Sakamaki T, et al. Classification of sensitive skin and development of treatment system appropriate for each group. IFSCC Mag. 2003;6:303-7.
11. Heughebaert C, Shalita A. Comedogenesis. In: Shalita AR, Del Rosso JQ, Webster GF, editors. Acne vulgaris. New York: Informa; 2011. pp. 28-42.

12. Baumann L. Sensitive skin. In: Baumann L, editor. Cosmetic dermatology. Mc Graw Hill; 2009. p. 94-5.
13. Yamamoto A, Takenouchi, Ito M. Impaired water barrier function in acne vulgaris. Arch Dermatol Res. 1985;287:214-8.
14. Del Rosso JQ, Levin J. The clinical relevance of maintaining the functional integrity of the stratum corneum in both healthy and disease-affected skin. J Clin Aesthet Dermatol. 2011;4(9):22-42.
15. Kurokawa I, Mayer-da-Silva A, Gollnick H, et al. Monoclonal antibody labeling for cytokeratins and filaggrin in the human pilosebaceous unit of normal, seborrhoeic and acne skin. J Invest Dermatol. 1988:91:566-71.
16. Jarrousse V, Castex-Rizzi N, Khammari A, et al. Modulation of integrins and filaggrin expression by Propionibacterium acnes extracts on keratinocytes. Arch Dermatol Res. 2007;299:441-7.
17. Common JE, Brown SJ, Haines RL, et al. Filaggrin null mutations are not a protective factor for acne vulgaris. J Invest Dermatol. 2011;131(6):1378-80.
19. Zaenglein AL, Thiboutot DM. Acne vulgaris. In: Bolognia J, Jorrizo JL, Schaffer JV, (Eds). Dermatology. Spain: Elsevier-Saunders; 2012. p. 545-58.
20. Kircik LH. Microsphere technology: hype or help? J Clin Aesthet Dermatol. 2011;4(5):27-31.
21. Weber ST, Thiele JJ, Han N, et al. Topical alpha-tocotrienol supplementation inhibits lipid peroxidation but fails to mitigate increased transepidermal water loss after benzoyl peroxide treatment to human skin. Free Radical Biol Med. 2003;34(2):170-6.
22. Thiboutot D, Del Rosso JQ. Acne vulgaris and the epidermal barrier: Is acne vulgaris associated with inherent epidermal abnormalities that cause impairment of barrier functions? Do any topical acne therapies alter the structural and/or functional integrity of the epidermal barrier? J Clin Aesthet Dermatol. 2013;6(2):18-24.
23. Tagami H. Location-related differences in structure and function of the stratum corneum with special emphasis on facial skin. Int J Cosmet Sci. 2008;30:413-34.
24. Feldman SR, Chen DM. How patients experience and manage dryness and irritation from acne treatment. J Drugs Dermatol. 2011;10(6):605-8.
25. Draelos ZD, Ertel KD, Berge CA. Facilitating facial retinization through barrier improvement. Cutis. 2006;78:275-81.
26. Layton AM, Eady EA, Zouboulis CC. Acne. In: Griffiths C, Barker J, Bleiker T, editors. Rook's textbook of dermatology. UK: Blackwell Publishing; 2016. p. 90-9.
27. Del Rosso JQ. Topical antibiotics. In: Shalita AR, Del Rosso JQ, Webster GF, editors. Acne vulgaris. London: Informa Healthcare; 2011:95-104.
28. Elias PM, Fritsch PO, Lampe M, et al. Retinoid effects on epidermal structure, differentiation, and permeability. Lab Invest. 1981;44(6):531-40.
29. Del Rosso JQ. Clinical relevance of skin barrier changes associated with the use of oral isotretinoin: the importance of barrier repair therapy in patient management. J Drugs Dermatol. 2013;12(6):626-31.
30. Elias PM. Epidermal effects of retinoids: Supramolecular observations and clinical implications. J Am Acad Dermatol. 1986;15(4 Pt 2):797-809.

31. Del Rosso JQ. The role of skin care as an integral component in the management of acne vulgaris: Part 1: The Importance of Cleanser and Moisturizer Ingredients, Design, and Product Selection. J Clin Aesthet Dermatol. 2013;6(12):19-27.
32. Subramanyan K. Role of mild cleansing in the management of patient skin. Dermatol Ther. 2004;17(Suppl 1):26-34.
33. Ananthapadmanabhan KP, Moore DJ, Subramanyan K, et al. Cleansing without compromise: The impact of cleansers on the skin barrier and the technology of mild cleanser. Dermatol Ther. 2004;17:16-25.
34. Hawkins SS, Subramanyan K, Liu D, et al. Cleansing, moisturizing, and sun-protection regimens for normal skin, self-perceived sensitive skin, and dermatologist-assessed sensitive skin. Dermatol Ther. 2004;17(Suppl 1):63-8.
35. Mukhopadhya P. Cleansers and their role in various dermatological disorders. Indian J Dermatol. 2011;56(1):2-6.
36. Chularojanamontri L, Tuchinda P, Kulthanan K, et al. Moisturizers for acne: What are their constituents? J Clin Aesthet Dermatol. 2014;7(5):36-44.
37. Smith RN, Mann NJ, Braue A, et al. A low-glycemic-load diet improves symptoms in acne vulgaris patients: A randomized controlled trial. Am J Clin Nutr. 2007;86:107-15.

4
CHAPTER

Skin Care in Sensitive Skin of Rosacea

Karen Koch, Ncoza Dlova

INTRODUCTION

Rosacea is a common chronic inflammatory disorder affecting the face and eyes. It presents with a wide range of symptoms including erythema, telangiectasia, pustules, rhinophyma, and ocular irritation.

PATHOGENESIS

The exact pathogenesis is not clear and different subtypes of rosacea may have specific factors:
- Neurovascular dysregulation: Vasodilation leading to easy flushing and persistent erythema is easily triggered in rosacea. Abnormal receptors and vasoactive peptides are some of the proposed mechanisms[1]
- Ultraviolet (UV) light and heat: The role of UV light in rosacea is controversial. UV exposure may aggravate erythrotelangiectatic rosacea but not necessarily other subtypes[2]
- Immune dysregulation: Abnormal activation of antimicrobial peptide cathelicidin via toll-like receptors leads to an inflammatory cascade. Enzymes such as matrix metalloproteinases are found in increased concentrations in rosacea. They are thought to lead to chronic inflammation, hardening, and thickening of the skin[2,3]
- Microorganisms: Hypersensitivity to *Demodex folliculorum* mite is a known trigger for rosacea.[2] Other possible microbial organisms associated with rosacea include *Bacillus olenorium* (a bacteria

found within the *Demodex* mite), *Helicobacter pyloria*, and *Staphylococcus epidermidis*[4]
- Genetic predisposition: Family members have an increased risk of rosacea but the exact genetic basis has not been established.[5]

EPIDEMIOLOGY

The exact prevalence of rosacea is unknown but it is estimated to affect from 1–22% in fair-skinned individuals.[6,7] Adults over 30 are more commonly affected. Overall, women are more likely to be affected than men.[7]

CLINICAL PRESENTATION

The clinical presentation of rosacea is varied. Onset is usually over the age of 3.[7] Frequent or easy flushing or blushing may be one of the first symptoms of rosacea. Skin is usually sensitive and tends to be easily irritated by skin products. Flushing is aggravated by spicy food, alcohol, exercise, or UV exposure.

This is followed by persistent facial redness and fine telangiectasia, typically sparing the periocular and perioral region.

Rosacea may progress to papules and pustules without comedones affecting the nose, forehead, cheeks, and chin which is characteristic of rosacea. Pustules are dome-shaped rather than pointed.

The skin may also become flaky or thickened (due to underlying edema). The nose (rhinophyma), forehead (metophyma), and chin (gnathophyma) may become thickened and enlarge due to sebaceous hyperplasia.

Ocular rosacea accompanies 40% of facial rosacea but may occur in isolation. It is characterized by blepharitis. The eyes will feel gritty with papules, sores, styes (hordeolum) and telangiectasia along the eyelid margin.

Severe edema over the whole face may occur due to lymphatic obstruction (Morbihan disease).

"Skin sensitivity" is a frequent finding in rosacea and is characterized by irritation by hot water, acidic compounds (retinoic acid, lactic acid), soaps, and chemicals. It is important that the cosmetic and skincare product formulation considerations for rosacea patients include cosmetic products with minimal ingredients, lack of common sensitizers, least number of irritants, and absence of skin stimulants.[8]

Proper instructions and guidance on use of proper general skin care products (such as gentle cleansers, moisturizers, sun protection, and avoidance of triggers) is prudent for all rosacea patients, to ensure optimal treatment effects.

According to Schaller et al., the following skincare advice is recommended and crucial for rosacea patients, e.g., use of sunscreen (SPF 30+), frequent use of suitable nonirritating moisturizers and use of gentle over-the-counter cleansers.[9]

CLASSIFICATION/GRADING

The National Rosacea Society Expert Committee has divided up rosacea into the following subtypes:[10]
- Type I: Erythematotelangiectatic rosacea (ETR)—facial erythema, flushing, dryness, and increased overall skin sensitivity
- Type II: Papulopustular rosacea—papules and pustules occurring over the nose, cheeks, and forehead; may also have coexisting ETR
- Type III: Phymatous rosacea—thickened skin due to sebaceous hypertrophy leading to enlargement and distortion of the nose, forehead, chin, and ears
- Type IV: Ocular rosacea—increased eye sensitivity with inflammation of the eyelid margins. This results in redness, burning, tearing, and frequent hordeolum (stye) formation. Ocular rosacea is not always associated with cutaneous rosacea.

DIAGNOSIS

The diagnosis is usually made on history and clinical appearance.

HISTOPATHOLOGY

On biopsy, dilation of superficial vessels, perivascular and perifollicular lymphocytic, and neutrophilic infiltrates may be seen. Pustules will show neutrophilic collections in hair follicles. *Demodex* mites may be seen in dilated hair follicles.[11]

TREATMENT

General Measures for Sensitive Skin of Rosacea[9]

- Gentle skin care—avoid any harsh soaps, rubbing the skin, or enzymatic exfoliators
- Products—avoid oil-based cosmetics or facial products. Use of water-based products is advised
- Sun protection—advise use sunscreen with UVA and UVB protection (SPF ≥30). Avoid direct sun in peak hours
- Avoid irritating products—toners, astringents, alcohol-based skin products, or fragrances on the skin
- Camouflage—use face creams or powders that contain a green pigment base. This counteracts the overall redness of the skin. This is effective for both men and women
- Avoid triggers—avoid known triggers such as overheating, hot showers, steam rooms, spicy food, and alcohol should be avoided. Patients may benefit from keeping a diary to accurately identify triggers
- Review medications—nicotinic acid and vasodilators may exacerbate facial flushing.

Medications

The use of topical and oral medications to treat rosacea depends on the subtype and severity of disease. Patients often have more than one subtype of rosacea requiring combinations of treatments. Oral agents should be used in conjunction with appropriate topical treatments.

The ROSacea COnsensus (ROSCO) guidelines suggest a symptom-based algorithm.[9]

Topical Treatments

- Topical brimonidine: This is an α2-adrenergic receptor antagonist used for facial redness in ETR type rosacea. It is applied once daily with onset within 30 minutes with effects lasting up to 12 hours.[4] There is a small risk of transient rebound erythema estimated to affect up to 20% of users.[12] The treatment is generally well-tolerated with few patients reporting burning, stinging, and a contact dermatitis

- Topical oxymetazoline: This is an α1 and partial α2-adrenergic receptor antagonist approved in 2017 by the FDA for facial erythema in rosacea. The onset of effect is within 3 hours and the reduction in redness lasts up to 12 hours. Potential side effects include skin irritation, pain, and pruritus
- Topical azelaic acid: Azelaic acid has anti-inflammatory and antioxidative qualities. It is useful in the treatment of platelet-rich plasma (PRP) rosacea. The exact mechanism of action is not known but it is thought to reduce cathelicidin production. Twice daily use of azelaic acid has been shown to be at least as effective as topical metronidazole in treating rosacea.[13] Other studies suggest no significant difference between twice and once daily application.[14] Treatment may take a few weeks to show effect[6]
- Topical metronidazole: This antibiotic and antiprotozoal medication also has anti-inflammatory and antioxidant properties.[15] It is used to treat both PRP and ETR. Different formulations (cream, gel, and foam) have shown similar efficacy.[16] Onset of effect is usually seen within 2-4 weeks. Side effects that have been reported include burning, stinging, and dryness[16]
- Ivermectin 1% cream: Ivermectin is an antiparasite agent with anti-inflammatory properties. One of the mechanisms of action is its anti-*Demodex* effect on the skin. It is safe and well-tolerated. It has been shown to be effective at reducing pustular rosacea.[17] Compared to metronidazole, topical ivermectin has been shown to be more effective in treating inflammatory lesions[18]
- Other agents used in the treatment of rosacea for which there is less evidence include permethrin, clindamycin, azithromycin, benzoyl peroxide, tacrolimus, and pimecrolimus.[4]

Oral Medications

- Tetracyclines: Tetracycline, doxycycline, and minocycline are used in therapeutic and subantimicrobial doses to treat both telangiectatic and papulopustular rosacea. Tetracyclines have anti-inflammatory effects on the skin. Doxycycline in particular has been shown to be equally effective at a dose of 100 mg/day and 40 mg (slow release) per day.[19] Minocycline is less often used to the risk of adverse effects. The starting dose for doxycycline is 50-100 mg daily and for tetracycline 250-500 mg twice daily.

The Sensitive Skin: Treatment Modalities and Cosmeceuticals

Treatment needs to be continued for at least 4–12 weeks to maximize effectiveness. Tetracyclines should not be used in children under the age of 9 years
- Macrolides: Clarithromycin at a dosage of 250 mg twice daily for one month followed by 250 mg daily for a month showed similar efficacy to doxycycline and may be a useful alternative for patients who cannot tolerate tetracyclines[20]
- Isotretinoin: Isotretinoin is a vitamin A derivative retinoid with anti-inflammatory properties. It effectively reduces the size of enlarged sebaceous glands and decreases sebum production. It is particularly useful for resistant papulopustular type rosacea and inflammatory phase rhinophyma. It can be associated with significant side effects. Most notably it is highly teratogenic. Fertile female patients are advised to use two forms of contraceptive throughout its use and one month after stopping treatment. Baselines screening for pregnancy, liver function, and triglycerides should be done. The recommended dosage to treat rosacea is 0.3 mg/kg/day for at least 3 months.[21]

Light and Laser Therapy

Treatment with light-based is particularly used to target erythema and telangiectasia. During treatment, energy is absorbed by hemoglobin within vessels leading to coagulation. Commonly used forms of laser include: Intense-pulsed-light (500–1,200 nm), potassium titanyl phosphate (KTP, 532 nm) and pulsed dye laser (585–595 nm).[22,23] Treatment may be effective but do not cure the condition. Retreatment is generally required.[24]

Cosmeceuticals

There is an increased interest in natural ingredients to reduce irritation and inflammation of rosacea. Some of these ingredients include licorice, chamomile, turmeric, niacinamide, teas, colloidal oatmeal, quassia amara extract and eperua falcata bark extract.[4,25]

CONCLUSION

Rosacea is a common multifactorial skin condition that primarily affects women over the age of 30 years. Localised persistent facial flushing, papulopustules and general skin sensitivity often leads to social embarrassment. Overall skin sensitivity means that commonly used skin care products can aggravate the condition. Education, avoidance of triggers, cosmetic camouflage and appopriate medical treatments can greatly enhance the quality of life of patients with rosacea.

REFERENCES

1. Aubdool AA, Brain SD. Neurovascular aspects of skin neurogenic inflammation. J Investig Dermatol Symp Proc. 2011;15(1):33-9.
2. Crawford GH, Pelle MT, James WD. Rosacea: I. Etiology, pathogenesis, and subtype classification. J Am Acad Dermatol. 2004;51(3):327-41.
3. Yamasaki K, Gallo RL. The molecular pathology of rosacea. J Dermatol Sci. 2009;55(2):77-81.
4. Weinkle AP, Doktor V, Emer J. Update on the Management of Rosacea. Plast Surg Nurs. 2015;35(4):184-202.
5. Abram K, Silm H, Maaroos HI, Oona M. Risk factors associated with rosacea. J Eur Acad Dermatol Venereol. 2010;24(5):565-71.
6. Elewski BE, Draelos Z, Dreno B, et al. Rosacea - global diversity and optimized outcome: proposed international consensus from the Rosacea International Expert Group. J Eur Acad Dermatol Venereol. 2011;25(2):188-200.
7. Tan J, Berg M. Rosacea: current state of epidemiology. J Am Acad Dermatol. 2013;69(6 Suppl 1):S27-35.
8. Draelos ZD. Sensitive skin: perceptions, evaluation, and treatment. Am J Contact Dermat. 1997;8(2):67-78.
9. Schaller M, Almeida LM, Bewley A, et al. Rosacea treatment update: recommendations from the global ROSacea COnsensus (ROSCO) panel. Br J Dermatol. 2017;176(2):465-71.
10. Wilkin J, Dahl M, Detmar M, et al. Standard classification of rosacea: Report of the National Rosacea Society Expert Committee on the Classification and Staging of Rosacea. J Am Acad Dermatol. 2002;46(4):584-7.
11. Marks R, Harcourt-Webster JN. Histopathology of rosacea. Arch Dermatol. 1969;100(6):683-91.
12. Docherty JR, Steinhoff M, Lorton D, et al. Multidisciplinary Consideration of Potential Pathophysiologic Mechanisms of Paradoxical Erythema with Topical Brimonidine Therapy. Adv Ther. 2016;33(11):1885-95.
13. Elewski BE, Fleischer AB Jr, Pariser DM. A comparison of 15% azelaic acid gel and 0.75% metronidazole gel in the topical treatment of papulopustular rosacea: results of a randomized trial. Arch Dermatol. 2003;139(11):1444-50.
14. Thiboutot DM, Fleischer AB Jr, Del Rosso JQ, et al. Azelaic acid 15% gel once daily versus twice daily in papulopustular rosacea. J Drugs Dermatol. 2008;7(6):541-6.
15. Miyachi Y. Potential antioxidant mechanism of action for metronidazole: implications for rosacea management. Adv Ther. 2001;18(6):237-43.

16. Wolf JE Jr, Del Rosso JQ. The CLEAR trial: results of a large community-based study of metronidazole gel in rosacea. Cutis. 2007;79(1):73-80.
17. Stein L, Kircik L, Fowler J, et al. Efficacy and safety of ivermectin 1% cream in treatment of papulopustular rosacea: results of two randomized, double-blind, vehicle-controlled pivotal studies. J Drugs Dermatol. 2014;13(3):316-23.
18. Taieb A, Ortonne JP, Ruzicka T, et al. Superiority of ivermectin 1% cream over metronidazole 0.75% cream in treating inflammatory lesions of rosacea: a randomized, investigator-blinded trial. Br J Dermatol. 2015;172(4):1103-10.
19. Webster GF. An open-label, community-based, 12-week assessment of the effectiveness and safety of monotherapy with doxycycline 40 mg (30-mg immediate-release and 10-mg delayed-release beads). Cutis. 2010;86(5 Suppl):7-15.
20. Torresani C, Pavesi A, Manara GC. Clarithromycin versus doxycycline in the treatment of rosacea. Int J Dermatol. 1997;36(12):942-6.
21. Sbidian E, Vicaut E, Chidiack H, et al. A Randomized-Controlled Trial of Oral Low-Dose Isotretinoin for Difficult-To-Treat Papulopustular Rosacea. J Invest Dermatol. 2016;136(6):1124-9.
22. Papageorgiou P, Clayton W, Norwood S, et al. Treatment of rosacea with intense pulsed light: significant improvement and long-lasting results. Br J Dermatol. 2008;159(3):628-32.
23. Alam M, Dover JS, Arndt KA. Treatment of facial telangiectasia with variable-pulse high-fluence pulsed-dye laser: comparison of efficacy with fluences immediately above and below the purpura threshold. Dermatol Surg. 2003;29(7):681-4.
24. Clark SM, Lanigan SW, Marks R. Laser treatment of erythema and telangiectasia associated with rosacea. Lasers Med Sci. 2002;17(1):26-33.
25. Emer J, Waldorf H, Berson D. Botanicals and anti-inflammatories: natural ingredients for rosacea. Semin Cutan Med Surg. 2011;30(3):148-55.

CHAPTER 5

Topical Steroid Damaged/Dependent Face

Yasmeen J Bhat, Safia Bashir

INTRODUCTION

Topical corticosteroids are undoubtedly the most important drugs in a dermatologist's armamentarium. The introduction of topical steroids into dermatologic therapy in 1952 was probably one of the most important milestones, owing to their potent anti-inflammatory and antiproliferative effects.[1] Soon afterwards, the adverse effects of topical corticosteroids were first reported in 1955.[2] The misuse of topical corticosteroids over the years, with failure to follow proper guidelines for their use both by medical practitioners and patients led to a plethora of cutaneous and systemic adverse effects of these drugs. The local adverse effects of topical steroids were, however, far more prevalent than the systemic ones.[3,4] It was later in 1970s that the addictive potential of topical corticosteroids was recognized.[5,6] Chronic misuse of these drugs led to psychological and physical dependence on them. The face was the most common site of this "addiction." In subsequent years, other terms like "dermatitis rosaciformis steroidica,"[7] "red skin syndrome,"[8] and "steroid induced rosacea like dermatitis"[9] were used for the condition that affects the facial skin due to chronic misuse of topical corticosteroids.

The term "topical steroid damaged/dependent face (TSDF)" was coined by Koushik Lahiri (India) in March 2008 and may be defined as "*the semipermanent or permanent damage to the skin of the face precipitated by the irrational, indiscriminate, unsupervised, or prolonged use of topical corticosteroids resulting in a plethora of cutaneous signs and symptoms and psychological dependence on the drug.*"[10]

PATHOGENESIS

Although the exact pathogenesis is not known, some of the postulated mechanisms for the occurrence of TSDF include:[11]
- Effect of topical corticosteroids on "skin immune system": Topical corticosteroid induced chronic immunosuppression and the release of proinflammatory cytokines in the skin may be responsible for some of the manifestations of TSDF
- Effect on cutaneous blood vessels (role of nitric oxide): Prolonged use of topical corticosteroids on the face leads to suppression of endothelium derived relaxing factor, nitric oxide being the most important among them. The suppression of nitric oxide release leads to sustained vasoconstriction with accumulation of this nitric oxide. However, on temporary withdrawal of topical steroids, vasodilation occurs leading to symptoms of erythema, itching, and burning. Reuse of topical corticosteroids to suppress these symptoms again leads to vasoconstriction. This cycle of repeated vasoconstriction/vasodilation known as the trampoline effect/neon sign leads to a build up of nitric oxide and continues until a physiologic response ensues, which causes the cutaneous vasculature to become fully dilated (even beyond the initial presteroid diameter) due to the accumulated nitric oxide
- Effects on pituitary adrenal axis—suppression of the axis.

CLINICAL PRESENTATION

The signs and symptoms of TSDF may present after prolonged topical corticosteroid use or may become evident as a rebound phenomenon once the offending topical steroid is discontinued.
Various manifestations of TSDF include:
- Erythema: Erythema may be considered as the hallmark manifestation of TSDF. This becomes more evident after total withdrawal of the topical corticosteroid. It is usually accompanied by a burning sensation which may be mild or severe. The erythema, however, resolves within 2 weeks only to reappear within a few days. Patients continue to develop intermittent flares of erythema which may spread beyond the area of initial corticosteroid application or even to distant sites.[8] In severe cases, erythema may be accompanied by edema or

vesiculation.[8] Dryness, scaling, and itching may accompany the resolving phase
- Telangiectasia: Abnormal dilatation of capillaries due to stimulation of nitric oxide release from endothelial cells of dermal vessels during withdrawal phase leads to telangiectasia
- Papulopustular lesions and acneiform eruption: These may be attributed to the degradation of follicular epithelium caused by topical corticosteroids with resultant extrusion of follicular contents.[12] Topical steroids also induce comedone formation by rendering the follicular epithelium more responsive to comedogenesis.[13,14] Overgrowth of microorganisms due to cutaneous immunosuppression may present as inflammatory papules and pustules (Fig. 1)[15]
- Atrophy: Atrophy is commonly seen in patients with topical steroid abuse in the form of increased transparency and shininess of skin. This occurs not only because of the suppressive effects of topical corticosteroids on cell proliferation but also due to decreased fibroblast growth and reduced synthesis of collagen and acid mucopolysaccharides (Fig. 2)[16]

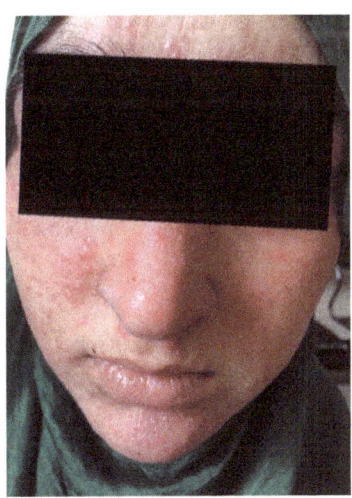

FIG. 1: Acneiform eruption in a patient with chronic steroid abuse.
(For color version, see Plate 1)

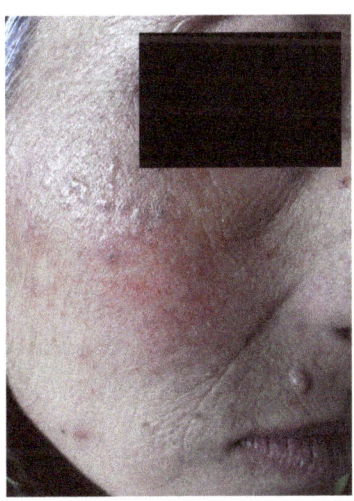

FIG. 2: Atrophy, telangiectasia, and comedones in topical steroid damaged/dependent face.
(For color version, see Plate 2)

- Hypopigmentation and hyperpigmentation: While the mechanism of topical corticosteroid induced hyperpigmentation remains largely unknown, hypopigmentation due to topical corticosteroids may be induced by inhibition of prostaglandin or cytokine production in various epidermal cells by topical steroids leading to an altered melanocyte function by suppression of secretory metabolic products from melanocytes.[17] These pigmentary alterations generally improve once the patient stops using topical corticosteroids
- Hirsutism: While hirsutism is a more common manifestation of systemic steroid use, many patients with TSDF tend to have abnormal facial hair growth
- Rosacea and perioral dermatitis: Features of rosaceiform and perioral dermatitis are seen in patients with chronic abuse of potent topical corticosteroids. A significantly increased density of *Demodex folliculorum* was reported by Bonnar et al. in patients with steroid induced rosacea (Figs 3 and 4)[18]
- Other features: In addition, patients with TSDF often present with features like photosensitivity, tinea incognito (Fig. 5), and allergic contact dermatitis.

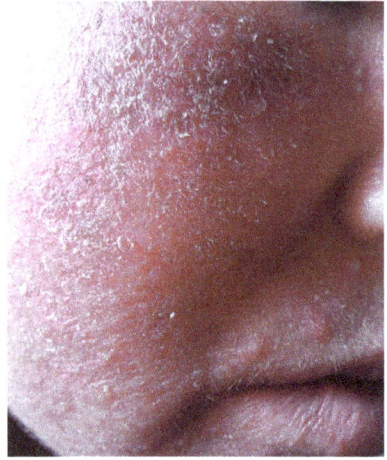

FIG. 3: Rosacea-like features in a patient with history of prolonged application of betamethasone valerate on face.
(For color version, see Plate 2)

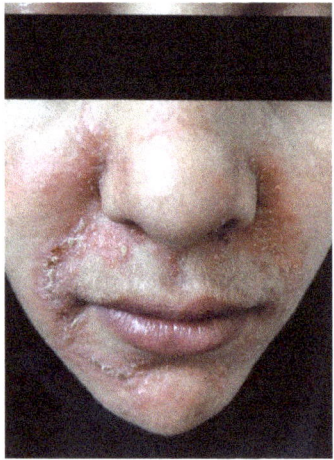

FIG. 4: Topical steroid damaged/dependent face presenting as perioral dermatitis.
(For color version, see Plate 2)

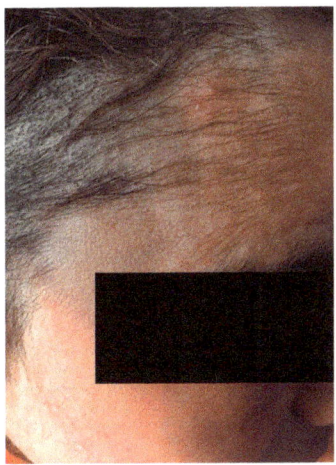

FIG. 5: Tinea incognito in a patient with chronic steroid abuse. *(For color version, see Plate 2)*

DERMOSCOPIC FEATURES OF TOPICAL STEROID DAMAGED/DEPENDENT FACE (FIGS 6–9)

Various features demonstrated by dermoscopy in TSDF include:
- Linear, tortuous, and polygonal vessels
- Red diffuse areas
- Atrophic areas, white structureless areas, or patches between vessels
- White hairs derived from hypertrichosis.

Status Cosmeticus

The term has been used to describe a condition in patients with chronic topical steroid abuse who are unable to tolerate any form of makeup or cosmetic application to the face; which results in immediate erythema and burning sensation. Atrophy, telangiectasia, and acneiform eruption are usually observed on the face in these patients.

MANAGEMENT OF TOPICAL STEROID DAMAGED/DEPENDENT FACE

The management of TSDF is difficult and requires a lot of patience on part of the patient as well as the treating dermatologist. There is no

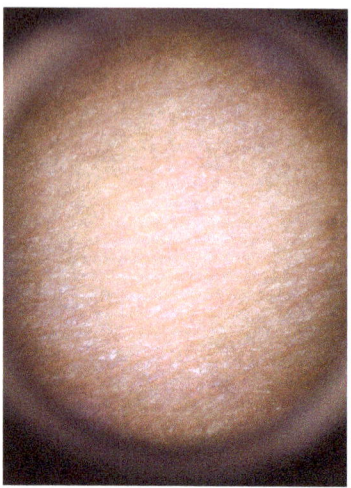

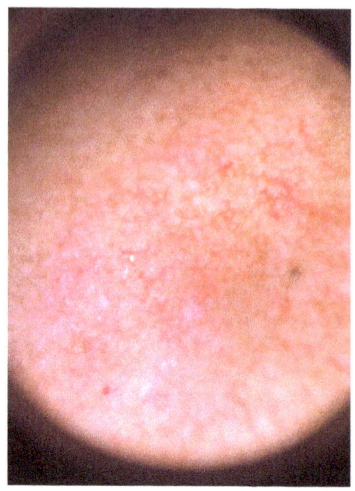

FIG. 6: Dermoscopic appearance of atrophic facial skin following topical steroid abuse (nonpolarized mode). *(For color version, see Plate 3)*

FIG. 7: Irregular, branching and polygonal vessels with structureless areas in between (polarized mode). *(For color version, see Plate 3)*

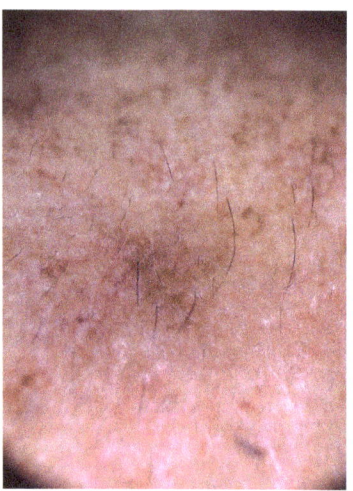

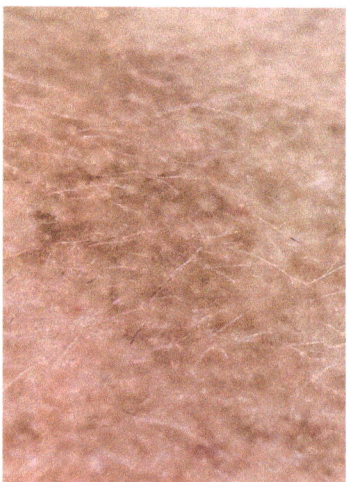

FIG. 8: Tortuous vessels, perifollicular hypopigmentation, and brown clods (polarized mode). *(For color version, see Plate 3)*

FIG. 9: Hypertrichosis presenting as light colored hair, arcuate pigmentation (polarized mode). *(For color version, see Plate 3)*

single drug which is effective in all patients and treatment needs to be tailored according to the varying presentations of the condition.

While some physicians advocate shifting the patients to less potent preparations before withdrawing the topical corticosteroid,[9] others are in favor of complete cessation of corticosteroids usage on first contact with the affected patient. Using less potent topical steroids may help patients to cope better with the withdrawal symptoms especially in those who are unable to tolerate the flares. Total cure of the condition is expected in 6–24 months (with intermittent flares and remissions) without the use of any medication once the topical steroids are withdrawn.[8]

Various treatment modalities that have been tried in patients with TSDF include:

- Antibiotics: Oral antibiotics like tetracycline, doxycycline, minocycline, and azithromycin may be effective in patients with papulopustular lesions, perioral dermatitis, and rosacea-like features.[19] In addition, topical metronidazole has also been found effective in some cases[20]
- Topical calcineurin inhibitors: Various studies have shown the efficacy of topical calcineurin inhibitors like tacrolimus and pimecrolimus during the withdrawal phase in TSDF and they appear to decrease the time taken for complete resolution of symptoms (Figs 10 and 11)[19,21,22]

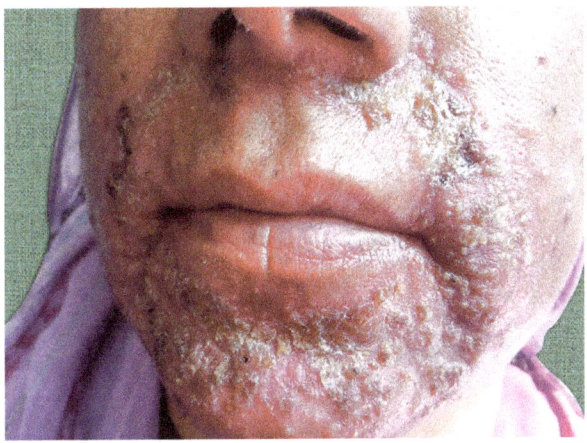

FIG. 10: Perioral dermatitis in a patient with chronic steroid abuse. *(For color version, see Plate 4)*

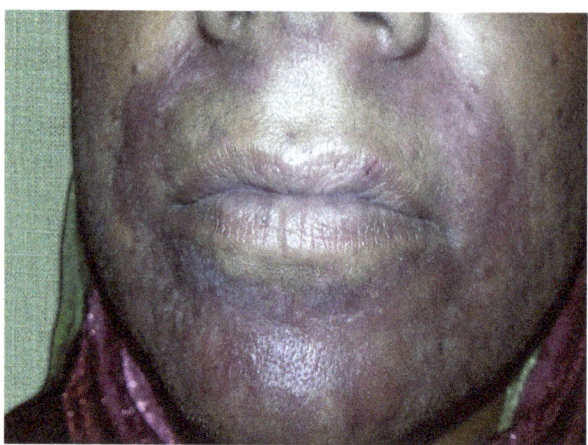

FIG. 11: Excellent response of perioral dermatitis to topical tacrolimus. *(For color version, see Plate 4)*

- Alpha-adrenergic agonists: Topical xylometazoline which acts by directly constricting the cutaneous vasculature thereby reducing the erythema and flushing in TSDF has been recently proposed as a treatment option in TSDF[23]
- Others measures: Cold compresses may help in relieving erythema and burning sensation during acute flares. Soap free cleansers, emollients, calamine, and oral and topical vitamin C and E may improve therapeutic outcome in patients with TSDF.[19] Intense pulsed light has also been tried.

CONCLUSION

Topical corticosteroids are immensely valuable in treating a wide spectrum of dermatological diseases owing to their anti-inflammatory, antiproliferative, and immunosuppressive properties. However, repeated or prolonged application of topical corticosteroids on face leads to epidermal atrophy, degeneration of dermal structure, and collagen deterioration over time. The resulting condition (TSDF) because of being so difficult to treat can pose a serious psychological burden to the patient and can be equally frustrating to the treating dermatologist. Drugs like topical calcineurin inhibitors and alpha-adrenergic agonists have shown some promise in recent studies in the management of TSDF. The need to create public awareness regarding the potential adverse effects of self use of potent topical corticosteroids on face and to stop the easy and over the counter availability of potent topical steroids cannot be emphasized enough.

REFERENCES

1. Smith EW. Do we need new and different glucocorticoids? A re-appraisal of the various congeners and potential alternatives. Curr Probl Dermatol. 1993;21:1-10.
2. Fitzpatrick TB, Griswold HC, Hicks JH. Sodium retention and edema from percutaneous absorption of fludrocortisones acetate. J Am Med Assoc. 1955;158:1149-52.
3. Robertson DB, Maibach HI. Topical corticosteroids. Int J Dermatol. 1982;21:59-67.
4. Lagos BR, Maibach HI. Frequency of application of topical corticosteroids: An overview. Br J Dermatol. 1998;139:763-6.
5. Burry JN. Topical drug addiction: Adverse effects of fluorinated corticosteroid creams and ointments. Med J Aust. 1973;1:393-6.
6. Kligman AM. Letter: Topical steroid addicts. JAMA. 1976;235:1550.
7. Basta Juzbasic A, Subic JS, Ljubojevic S. Demodex folliculorum in development of dermatitis rosaceiformis steroidica and rosacea-related diseases. Clin Dermatol. 2002;20:135-40.
8. Rapaport MJ, Rapaport V. The red skin syndromes: Corticosteroid addiction and withdrawal. Expert Rev Dermatol. 2006;1:547-61.
9. Rathi SK, Kumrah L. Topical corticosteroid-induced rosacea-like dermatitis: A clinical study of 110 cases. Indian J Dermatol Venereol Leprol. 2011;77:42-6.
10. Lahiri K, Coondoo A. Topical steroid damaged/dependent face (TSDF): An entity of cutaneous pharmacodependence. Indian J Dermatol. 2016;61:265-72.
11. Rapaport MJ, Lebwohl M. Corticosteroid addiction and withdrawal in the atopic: The red burning skin syndrome. Clin Dermatol. 2003;21:201-14.
12. Hengge UR, Ruzicka T, Schwartz RA, et al. Adverse effects of glucocorticosteroids. J Am Acad Dermatol. 2006;54(1):1-15.
13. Kuflik JH, Schwartz RA. Acneiform eruptions. Cutis. 2000;66:97-100.
14. Momin S, Peterson A, Del Rosso JQ. Drug-induced acneform eruptions: Definitions and causes. Cosmet Dermatol. 2009;22:28-37.
15. Ghosh A, Sengupta S, Coondoo A, et al. Topical corticosteroid addiction and phobia. Indian J Dermatol. 2014;59:465-8.
16. Lavker RM, Schechter NM, Lazarus GS. Effects of TCS on human dermis. Br J Dermatol. 1986;115:101-7.
17. Friedman SJ, Butler DF, Pittelkow MR. Perilesional linear atrophy and hypopigmentation after intralesional corticosteroid therapy. Report of two cases and review of the literature. J Am Acad Dermatol. 1988;19:537-41.
18. Bonnar E, Eustace P, Powell FC. The Demodex mite population in rosacea. J Am Acad Dermatol. 1993;28(3):443-8.

19. Bhat YJ, Manzoor S, Qayoom S. Steroid-induced rosacea: A clinical study of 200 patients. Indian J Dermatol. 2011;56:30-2.
20. Ljubojeviae S, Basta-JuzbaSiae A, Lipozeneiae J. Steroid dermatitis resembling rosacea: Aetiopathogenesis and treatment. J Eur Acad Dermatol Venereol. 2002;16:121-6.
21. Goldman D. Tacrolimus ointment for the treatment of steroid-induced rosacea: A preliminary report. J Am Acad Dermatol. 2001;44:995-8.
22. Chu CY. An open-label pilot study to evaluate the safety and the efficacy of topically applied pimecrolimus cream for the treatment of steroid-induced rosacea-like eruption. J Eur Acad Dermatol Venereol. 2007;21:484-90.
23. Kakkar S, Sharma PK. Topical steroid-dependent face: Response to xylometazoline topical. Indian J Drugs Dermatol. 2017;3:87-9.

CHAPTER 6

Skin Care in Dermatitis and Psoriasis in Patients with Sensitive Skin

Ambika Damodaran, Trilokraj Tejasvi

INTRODUCTION

Sensitive skin is defined as a sensory reaction triggered by contactors and/or environmental factors, usually without a visible clinical manifestation. This condition is usually self-diagnosed due to development of symptoms within minutes to hours after contact with the stimulant and typically without obvious physical signs of irritation. The number of individuals with sensitivity is steadily increasing due to increase in the number of consumer products.[1] Patients with sensitive skin could also develop autoimmune conditions like psoriasis, atopic dermatitis (AD), and seborrheic dermatitis. In fact, significant proportion of patients with AD may complain about sensitive skin.

EPIDEMIOLOGY

Numerous host factors, environmental factors, and structural factors play a role in sensitive skin. Young adults aged between 18 and 50 years have more sensitive skin than the elderly. Women are more prone than men to sensitive skin due to the hormonal differences and the thinner epidermis. Current studies from the United Kingdom, North America, and other European countries show a high prevalence rate in women 51.4% versus 38.2% in men. Racial difference in the structure of the skin is associated with sensitive skin. Asians and African Americans have greater propensity to develop sensitive skin due to higher baseline transepidermal water loss (TEWL), a test to detect the barrier function. Caucasians have higher sensitivity to capsaicin followed by Asians and African Americans. Some pre-existing skin disorders such as AD, seborrheic dermatitis, and rosacea have also been linked to sensitive skin.[2,3] Currently, there are no epidemiological studies for evaluating the prevalence of sensitive skin in patients with psoriasis. There are few studies which have demonstrated a positive association between patients with AD and increased skin sensitivity. Few studies also suggest that patients with sensitive skin have a higher chance of developing contact dermatitis and there are others studies which refute this claim.[2]

RISK FACTORS

The face is the most common site for skin sensitivity probably due to the number of products used on the face, thinner barrier, and maximum number of nerve endings. Daily use of topical steroids can make the skin fragile and increase the risk of sensitivity. The nasolabial fold, malar eminences, chin, and upper lip are the most sensitive areas on the face. Skin on the scalp is also a common site for sensitivity. Other areas include volar aspect of the forearm, hands, and genital region. Women prone for sensitivity are also prone to have vulvar erythema. Sociocultural factors like diet, use of hygiene products like douches, perfumes, medications, and contraceptives can increase vulvar irritation.[3] The morphological presentation of psoriasis or eczema at these sites is a challenge toward making a diagnosis and management. Environmental factors such as cold, dry air in a winter climate, stress, air conditioners, pollution, heat, and sun exposure can trigger sensitive skin.[2,3]

PATHOPHYSIOLOGY

Pathophysiology of sensitive skin is not completely understood. The main hypothesis is attributed to changes observed in the stratum corneum which do not have an immunologic or allergic origin. There is an inverse relation between corneal thickness and skin permeability. Decrease in corneal thickness increases permeation of substances capable of inducing the release of cytokines, leukotrienes, and prostaglandins which in turn helps in the formation of neurotransmitters that stimulate nerve endings.[3]

Increased TEWL, decrease in ceramide, and decreased capacitance has also been observed in sensitive skin. Thus, adequate hydration, use of moisturizers, and emollients has showed to improve symptoms. Pre-existing skin conditions like atopy, seborrheic dermatitis, and rosacea alter the epidermal barrier and increase vascularity which aid in increasing the sensitivity of the skin.[4]

Other evidence observed is the alteration in the sensorineural function of cutaneous nerves. Increase in sensorineural activity is perceived as an unpleasant sensation in sensitive individuals. These are mediated through unmyelinated C fibers. The neurotransmitters like substance P, calcitonin gene related peptide induce vasodilation and degranulation of mast cells. Studies have also demonstrated the presence of neurosensory receptors like endothelin receptors, transient receptor potential family receptors (TRP) (noxious pain receptors), heat and cold receptors, and neurotropin receptors are expressed on nerve ending and keratinocytes. This may explain the response of sensitive skin toward different environmental, physical, and chemical factors. Endothelin receptors may be involved in mediating nociceptive symptoms in sensitive skin. Heat receptor TRPV1 (transient receptor potential vanilloid-1) is involved in epidermal barrier homeostasis. Cold receptor TRPM8 (transient receptor potential melastatin-8) is involved in cold mediated sensitive skin. Interaction of the physical factors with the neurosensory receptor may induce hypersensitivity and the symptoms of sensitive skin.[5-8]

Discussion regarding pathophysiology and genetics of psoriasis or AD is beyond the scope of this chapter. Studies have been shown that there is a compromised epidermal barrier function in psoriatic and atopic skin. In a recent study, evaluating barrier function of psoriatic skin showed significantly increased TEWL, and significantly decreased stratum corneum hydration, natural moisturizing factor (NMF), and free fatty acids in the involved skin when compared with uninvolved and normal skin. The TEWL and stratum corneum hydration returned to normal levels following clinical improvement of the lesion. This study showed that barrier function is defective in psoriasis skin. In another study evaluating the barrier function and repair in psoriatic skin showed that the barrier function is defective but the barrier repair mechanism is fully operational.[9,10]

Atopic dermatitis is an inflammatory disease due to loss of function mutation in filaggrin, a protein which contributes to form the NMF of the skin. It is well established by numerous studies that patients with AD have increased TEWL and has no correlation with stratum corneum thickness in contrast to normal controls. In one study, the observation was that even the uninvolved skin in patients with AD have a reduced epidermal barrier. Increased TEWL that arise from defective barrier results in opening the epidermal and dermal milieu to the antigens and thus, stimulating the cytokine release and the inflammatory cascade. This process would worsen the itch scratch cycle, barrier damage, increased antigen adsorption, and cutaneous hypersensitivity. In environmental induced dermatitis, xerosis, and surfactant induced scaly skin are associated with impaired barrier function, which includes reduction in NMF and change in stratum corneum lipids.[11]

CLINICAL FEATURES

The clinical symptoms of sensitive skin includes burning, pruritus, and tingling. There are no specific cutaneous signs of sensitive skin, they may present with nonspecific erythema, xerosis, desquamation, urticarial, and telangiectases. It is essential to thoroughly question the patient regarding cosmetic intolerance, personal, family, and occupational history. Complete examination for any signs and features of inflammation should be documented.

Patients with classic atopic eczema or dermatitis present with itchy, mild scaly patches to crusted plaques on flexural aspects of extremities often associated with diffuse xerosis, icthyosis, and hyperlinear palms. They also have propensity to develop contact dermatitis and secondary infection in form impetiginization. Based on chronicity, one may develop lichenification and pruriginous changes with dyspigmentation. They also may suffer from asthma and seasonal allergies. For management purposes AD could be classified as mild, moderate, and severe based on body surface area (BSA) involvement.

Seborrheic dermatitis patients classically present with itchy, gray, dull colored, and superficial scales on the scalp. Severe forms include involvement with erythematous, scaly patches on the scalp, hair bearing areas of the face, paranasal areas, hair bearing areas of the chest and back.

Skin Care in Dermatitis and Psoriasis in Patients with Sensitive Skin

Psoriasis patients present with either limited disease or extensive disease, the classic disease is characterized by well defined, erythematous patches, and plaques involving extensor aspects of extremities. The disease is further classified based on the sites of involvement (e.g., inverse psoriasis, scalp psoriasis, etc.). For treatment purposes it is classified based on BSA, as mild, moderate, and severe involvement. The other forms of disease include pustular and erythrodermic forms.

Although, there are no specific features or unique cutaneous signs or symptoms that have been reported in patients of AD, environmental induced dermatitis, seborrheic dermatitis, and psoriasis with sensitive skin, but one can imagine that these patients would definitely have heightened symptoms due to compromised epidermal barrier.

TREATMENT

Specific systemic and biologic treatment of psoriasis, AD, and other dermatitis is beyond scope of this chapter. The following treatment and management recommendations are guidelines for patients with sensitive skin, who also suffer from psoriasis and eczema. Due to multifactorial nature of the sensitive skin no standardized treatment management algorithm has been established. Consider patch testing in patients with known history of contact dermatitis or sensitization. Controlling underlying dermatitis contributes to the improvement of sensitive skin. Educate the patient to discontinue all cosmetics. If they insist on getting back to use them, then introduce one cosmetic at time after the dermatitis has resolved and the sensitivity has improved. Educate patients to use physical sun protectors who complain of sun sensitiveness. The addition of anti-inflammatory compounds, antioxidants, and specific vanilloid has shown to reduce inflammation and reduce vascular reactivity.

The TRPV1 plays a very important role in symptoms of sensitive skin, a selective inhibitor trans-4-tert-butylcyclohexanol has shown to inhibit the TRPV1; some medications are compounded with this molecule and are being used to treat sensitive skin. Another molecule, furocoumarin has shown to reduce pain related to this receptor in an experimental setting.[2,3]

Choosing the ideal topical medications is vital for the management of psoriasis and dermatitis patients with sensitive skin. The choice of the topical medications should be ointments over lotion or creams, as creams and alcohol based medications worsen the stinging or burning sensation. The other factors to consider are avoiding products which are unstable, have multiple unnecessary ingredients, and have common irritants and allergens.

Moisturizers are an important topical medication for management of both psoriasis and dermatitis and choosing the right one could be a challenge, especially in patients with sensitive skin. Following the below guidelines may be helpful for patients with sensitive skin. Studies have shown that adding moisturizers would reduce the use for topical steroids; moisturizers containing humectants like lactic acid, urea, pyrrolidone carboxylic acid, and preservatives like sorbic acid and benzoic acid are known to increase subjective sensations especially in patients with "status cosmeticus" who react to any product applied especially on the face. Fragrances and preservatives are identified as the common sensitizers; educate your patient to avoid moisturizers with fragrances. Propylene glycol is known to cause irritant and allergic contact dermatitis and also subjective or sensory irritation. Avoid moisturizers and topical medications that contain propylene glycol. Pure petrolatum or ceramide based lipid mixture that has shown to improve skin barrier and decrease TEWL. Pure petrolatum or ceramide based moisturizer would be an ideal moisturizer in patient with sensitive skin.[8,12]

Atopic Dermatitis

The keys to successful management of AD should include skin hydration and skin barrier repair, topical anti-inflammatory medications which include topical steroids and calcineurin inhibitors, control of infection and elimination of aggravating factors like allergens, irritants, and stress. These triggers could propagate the vicious itch scratch cycle in a patient with sensitive skin resulting in acute flares and ultimately, causing chronic changes like lichenification.

Use of calcineurin inhibitors and phototherapy could be tricky in patients with dermatitis. The most common side effect of topical calcineurin inhibitor is irritation, burning, and erythema. Patients should be educated about these side effects to improve compliance. Gradually escalating the strength of the calcineurin inhibitor and frequency of application could alleviate the symptoms. Similarly, educating the patient to use sun protectants during and after phototherapy may help their sun sensitivity.[2,3,8,12]

Psoriasis

For localized disease treatment with topical steroids (moderate to high potency) is the standard of care and the addition of moisturizers has been reported to reduce the need for application of topical steroids. In patients with sensitivity the general rule outlined above for choosing any kind of topical medications including moisturizers should be strictly followed. Studies have shown that artificial restoration of permeability barrier by occlusion has resulted in regression of lesions. Water in oil emollients have been reported to be as effective as steroid-sparing agents in plaque psoriasis and have shown to inhibit the development of Koebner response. One needs to be careful while choosing steroid sparing agents like vitamin D analogs, anthralin, or tar; as all of these compounds are irritants and could worsen the symptoms of sensitive skin. Educate the patients to use sun protective physical barriers on uninvolved skin to prevent exacerbation of symptoms during photo therapy and maintain adequate stratum corneum hydration via using topical moisturizers post-treatment. In patients with severe or erythrodermic psoriasis, management should include abundant moisturizers with topical steroids along with systemic or biologic therapy.[2,3,8,12]

CONCLUSION

Sensitive skin represents a widespread condition of susceptibility of exogenous and endogenous factors. An increase in skin permeability and altered nerve response is considered to be the cause of this sensitivity. Conditions like AD and psoriasis which compromise epidermal barrier could worsen the sensitive skin symptoms. Skin care in patients of psoriasis and dermatitis or eczema with sensitive skin could be very challenging, albeit the altered sensitivity is very prudent to treat the underlying dermatoses effectively so that the vicious cycle of itch scratch in AD or increased sensitivity in the form of burning, redness, and tingling can be tackled. Dermatologists and healthcare providers should be aware of patient skin sensitiveness while choosing the topical medications as this would promote compliance. Management should include patient education about their skin sensitiveness, the dos and don'ts, and adverse effects of various topical treatments.

REFERENCES

1. Ananthapadmanabhan KP, Moore DJ, Subramanyan K, et al. Cleansing without compromise: the impact of cleansers on the skin barrier and the technology of mild cleansing. Dermatologic Therapy. 2004;17:16-25.
2. Berardesca E, Farage M, Maibach H. Sensitive skin: An overview. Int J Cosmet Sci. 2013;35:2-8.
3. Duarte I, Silveira JE, Hafner M, et al. Sensitive skin: review of an ascending concept. Anais Brasileiros de Dermatologia. 2017:92(4):521-5.
4. Blattner C, Coman G, Blickenstaff N, et al. Percutaneous absorption of water in skin: A review. Rev Environ Health. 2014;29(3):175-80.
5. Goon AT, Yosipovitch G, Chan YH, et al. Barrier repair in chronic plaque-type psoriasis. Skin Res Technol. 2004;10:10-13.
6. Lee Y, Je YJ, Lee SS, et al. Changes in transepidermal water loss and skin hydration according to expression of aquaporin-3 in psoriasis. Ann Dermatol. 2012;24(2):16874.
7. Leung DY, Guttman-Yassky E. Deciphering the complexities of atopic dermatitis: Shifting paradigms in treatment approaches. J Allergy Clin Immunol. 2014;134(4):769-79.
8. Loden M. Role of topical emollients and moisturizers in the treatment of dry skin barrier disorders. Am J Clin Dermatol. 2003;4:771-88.
9. Rim JH, Jo SJ, Park JY, et al. Electrical measurement of moisturizing effects on skin hydration and barrier function in psoriasis patients. Clin Exp Dermatol. 2005;30:40913.
10. Takahashi H, Tsuji H, Minami-Hori M, et al. Defective barrier function accompanied by structural changes of psoriatic stratum corneum. J Dermatol. 2014;41:144-8.
11. Zaniboni MC, Samorano LP, Orfali RL, et al. Skin barrier in atopic dermatitis: Beyond filaggrin. An Bras Dermatol. 2016;91(4):472-8.
12. Eichenfield LF, Fowler JF Jr, Rigel DS, et al. Natural advances in eczema care. Cutis. 2007;80(6 Suppl):2-16

7
CHAPTER

Cosmetic Intolerance Syndrome

Surabhi Sinha

INTRODUCTION

The beauty industry is a $450 billion booming business, constantly being driven further up by the thirst for a perfect face and perfect skin, and more recently, the perfect selfie! New cosmetic products are continuously being introduced into the market, the consumers being spoilt for choice! With the increase in the number of cosmetics available, the number of adverse reactions too would be expected to go up. However, not all reactions would come to the notice of the dermatologist, as patients may change their product once they develop a reaction. Only when the reactions persist despite changing the product or if the patient cannot pinpoint the offender, will the dermatologist come into the picture. Hence, published literature is just skimming the tip of the iceberg, and adverse reactions to cosmetics may indeed be more prevalent, more so in the subset of people with sensitive skin.

Cosmetic intolerance syndrome (CIS) was first described by Maibach as an adverse skin reaction of individuals who are no longer able to tolerate a wide range of cosmetic products.[1,2] Fisher used the term "status cosmeticus" to describe one extreme of the CIS in which the individual gradually becomes completely intolerant to the application of any cosmetic product.[3]

Basically, it refers to a state of hyper-reactivity to environmental stimuli which would otherwise be innocuous. It may start with one or few cosmetics, but during the evolution of the disorder, the patient may become intolerant to any topically applied agent. Some patients may develop CIS over a period of time by overuse of skin toiletries like cleansers/toners or moisturizers, exfoliants, scrubs, and other cosmetics. Frequent use of these products may leave the skin of face vulnerable to sensitivity.

Cosmetic intolerance syndrome has been used interchangeably or as a part of the sensitive skin syndrome. Few of these patients have occult allergic contact/photoallergic contact dermatitis or contact urticaria, but the majority test negative for patch/photopatch tests or open/prick tests, respectively.[4]

It is now understood that most of these patients will fit the description of sensitive skin and need to be managed on similar lines with the focus on eliminating primarily cosmetics. Also, any cosmetic will be able to incite irritation on dermatitic skin so may not necessarily be included under the CIS.

FACTORS CONTRIBUTING TO ADVERSE REACTIONS TO COSMETIC PRODUCTS[5]

- Complexity of composition: One of the basic principles of "hypoallergenic" cosmetics is to keep the formula as simple as possible—the fewer the constituents, the lesser the chances of synergistic allergenicity and the easier it is to identify the offender
- Concentration of ingredients: Sensitization is concentration dependent to some extent, however, elicitation is not. Very low concentrations can trigger allergic contact dermatitis in previously sensitized individuals
- Purity: Impurities have been known to be allergenic e.g. in cocamidopropyl betaine
- Cosmetic ingredients in topical medications: Patients may become sensitized to an ingredient in a topical medication applied on diseased skin and later may develop reactions to cosmetics containing the same ingredient.

MANAGEMENT OF COSMETIC INTOLERANCE SYNDROME

The management hinges on "skin rest"—eliminating all possible topical agents whether the inciting agent has been identified or not.

Cosmetic Intolerance Syndrome

The "2 week strategy" described by Draelos is followed where all cosmetics, topical dermatologic products, over-the-counter medications are discontinued for 2 weeks at least. Visible sensitive skin will need appropriate treatment for 2 weeks or sometimes more. For invisible sensitive skin, the following are rough guidelines on which the management should be based:[1,6]

- Patch tests and photopatch tests to look for subclinical contact allergic/photocontact dermatitis in invisible sensitive skin
- Testing for contact urticaria
- Facial sting testing with 10% lactic acid to one nasolabial fold and normal saline to the other fold
- Only water/nonsoap cleansers to be used
- Allow the female patient to add one facial cosmetic at a time in the following order: Lipstick, face powder, and blush—one product in 2-4 weeks under careful supervision
- Use test cosmetics by applying them to a 2 cm area lateral to the eye for at least five consecutive nights. Cosmetics to be tested in the following order—mascara, eye-liner, eyebrow pencil, eye shadow, facial foundation, blush, facial powder, and any other colored facial cosmetic
- Use light nonocclusive make up and cosmetics
- Use cosmetics that have been tested for nickel and other heavy metals
- Use simple formulations (preferably less than 10 ingredients)
- Limited use of lip cosmetics can be considered safe unless lip symptoms exist
- Limited use of eye cosmetics to be allowed unless eyelid eczema exists
- Face powders are usually the safest form
- Glycerin plus rose water for moisturizing the face (if needed)
- Make a list of ingredients/products that the patient ought to avoid.

All these patients need to be evaluated and referred for signs of depression/dysmorphophobia/suicidal ideation. This subset of patients will need multidisciplinary approach. The future lies in "allergy apps"—wherein the application could analyze the cosmetic or makeup product with the help of just its bar code and could list out the ingredients and safer alternatives.

CONCLUSION

Cosmetic intolerance syndrome was described in association with facial cosmetics initially but now most patients will fit into the category of "Sensitive skin" and should be managed along similar lines. herbal and "hypoallergenic" products may not necessarily be safe and this should be reinforced with such patients.

REFERENCES

1. Maibach HI, Engasser PG. Dermatitis due to cosmetics. In: Fisher AA, editor. Contact Dermatitis. 3rd ed. Philadelphia: Lea & Febiger; 1986. pp. 368-82.
2. Maibach HI. The cosmetic intolerance syndrome. Ear Nose Throat J. 1987;66:29-33.
3. Fisher AA. Cutis. "Status cosmeticus": a cosmetic intolerance syndrome. Cutis. 1990;46:109-10.
4. Lachapelle JM, Maibach HI. Patch testing and prick testing: A practical guide. 1st ed. Berlin: Springer; 2003.
5. Goossens AE. Allergy and hypoallergenic products. In: Barel AO, Paye M, Maibach HI, editors. Handbook of cosmetic science & technology. 4th ed. USA: CRC Press; 2014.
6. Draelos ZD. Sensitive skin: Perceptions, evaluation and treatment. Am J Contact Dermat. 1997;8:67-78.

CHAPTER 8

Dermatological Products for Sensitive Skin: Practice Tips

Surabhi Sinha, Sidharth Tandon

INTRODUCTION

Sensitive skin as a condition has been defined more by the varied symptoms than by clinical signs or tests. It is associated with tightness, stinging, prickling, burning, tingling, or itching mainly on the face.[1] The condition is usually self-diagnosed and the role of an impaired barrier function or heightened neurosensory perception has been studied extensively in the causation of this protean entity.[2]

Various inciting factors have been implicated in its causation including environmental factors (extremes of weather conditions, ultraviolet radiation), chemical factors [facial exposure to harsh (low/high pH) soaps, long term corticosteroids, toiletries, pollutants], psychological stress, and hormonal influences.[1]

As a result of the vague and subjective symptoms, sensitive skin is a tough to manage condition for dermatologists. There is no single clinical or laboratory test to identify individuals with sensitive skin. Many tests have been used and are summarized in table 1.[3-6]

It is imperative to be aware of certain chemical ingredients in dermatological products that might precipitate the sensitivity or cause contact dermatitis in these patients. This chapter highlights practice tips for choosing safe and appropriate products for sensitive skin.

TABLE-1: Tests used to detect sensitive skin in individuals DMSO, dimethyl sulfoxide

Test	Method	Site	Result
Christensen and Kligman test[3]	Application of 10% racemic lactic acid in a hilltop chamber	Malar eminence	Divide stinging into mild, moderate, and severe and note the time for initial stinging
DMSO test[4]	Application of 90–100% dimethyl sulfoxide for 5 min	Forearm/cheek	Sensitive skin shows erythema/urticarial with burning
Sodium lauryl sulfate (SLS) occlusion test[5]	Application of various concentrations of SLS	Forearm	Erythema seen in sensitive skin
Lactic acid facial sting test[6]	Application of 10% lactic acid	Cheek/nasolabial folds	Stinging experienced by the patient rated on a scale of 1–4 at 2.5 and 5 min. Score of more than 3 seen in patients with sensitive skin

GENERAL GUIDELINES FOR TREATMENT OF SENSITIVE SKIN

- Moisturize. A good quality emollient is of utmost importance[7]
- Treat obvious dermatosis, if any, present ("visible" sensitive skin).[8] A 2-week course of a mild topical corticosteroid should usually suffice.
- Discontinue all topical applications for a period ranging from 2 weeks up to even 12 months in patients of "status cosmeticus" (See chapter on "Cosmetic Intolerance Syndrome").[8]

    Draelos et al., outlined the following guidelines for dermatological products to be used while treating a patient with sensitive skin:[9-11]

- Avoid substances testing positive on skin testing and other known irritant/allergic contaminants
- Avoid solvents like propylene glycol which enhance skin penetration and use polyethylene glycol instead
- Avoid volatile vehicles, vasodilatory substances, and sensory stimulants like methanol and camphor

Dermatological Products for Sensitive Skin: Practice Tips

- Use antioxidants
- Select low-sensitivity preservatives and surfactants. Products should contain preservatives to avoid formation of auto-oxidation by products. Paraben preservatives are preferred to formaldehyde and have been proven to be relatively safe despite the concerns around their use
- Products should be selected from a reputed manufacturer that uses pure ingredients free from contaminants.

CONTACT DERMATITIS DUE TO DERMATOLOGICAL PRODUCTS

Dermatological products might cause a variety of contact dermatitis reactions that would be more common and more severe in sensitive skin.[12] Patients may choose products labeled "for sensitive skin" or "hypoallergenic" because they believe these products will be gentle on their skin and less likely to cause an allergic reaction. However, because these terms are not regulated by the United States Food and Drug Administration, there is no guarantee that these products won't cause contact dermatitis.

Certain ingredients are more likely to cause the above mentioned reactions and hence, care should be taken during selection of the product in patients with sensitive skin. The reactions can be of the following types:
- Irritant contact dermatitis (ICD)
- Allergic contact dermatitis (ACD)
- Contact urticaria (CU)
- Photoallergic contact dermatitis (PACD)
- Phototoxic contact dermatitis (PTCD).

Irritant Contact Dermatitis

It is the most commonly encountered adverse reaction to dermatological products. It occurs due to stratum corneum (SC) damage without involvement of the immunologic system. The damage to the SC could occur due to very high/very low pH of the ingredients or volatile vehicles that dissolve the protective sebum or due to vigorous rubbing during topical application. Further, patients with "visible" sensitive skin, i.e., patients with atopic dermatitis, rosacea, xerotic eczema can develop ICD to most products due to their already impaired skin barrier. Patients complain of "skin allergy" to products which is usually not a true allergy but an ICD. The dermatitis should be resolved before the patients can apply cosmetics or dermatological products.

Allergic Contact Dermatitis

These reactions cannot be prevented by an intact SC. The only way to prevent it is avoidance of allergens. Most common ingredients causing ACD are as follows:[13]

- Fragrances (most common culprit): Linalool, limonene, hyxylcinnamal, and cinnamic aldehyde
- Preservatives: Quarternium-15, imidazolidinyl urea, diazolidinyl urea, bronopol and dimethyloldimethyl (DMDM) hydantoin (all formaldehyde-releasers) formaldehyde, methylparaben, butylparaben, propylparaben, methyldibromo glutaronitrile (MDBGN)
- P-phenylenediamine (PPD – in hair colors)
- Glyceryl thioglycolate (permanent wave solution component)
- Lanolin (emollient)
- Propylene glycol (organic solvent and humectant)
- Toluene sulfonamide/formaldehyde resin (nail polish component)
- Sunscreens: Most commonly benzophenones, dibenzoylmethanes, cinnamates. Benzophenone-3 is the leading allergen and photoallergen.

Contrary to expectations, fragrances are the most common allergens, outnumbering preservatives and PPD. Furthermore, under current labeling laws in most nations, manufacturers are permitted to use the term "fragrance-free" on products that include fragrance chemicals if those chemicals are utilized for another purpose (i.e., moisturizing) rather than changing the product's scent. Also, the term "unscented" may be used on products that utilize fragrances to mask a strong existing odor instead of creating a new scent. Thus, all products with the "fragrance free" label should not be considered safe.

Linalool, limonene, hyxylcinnamal and cinnamic aldehyde are the most frequent fragrances causing contact dermatitis.

The most common preservatives used are parabens (i.e., methylparaben, ethylparaben, propylparaben, butylparaben) and formaldehyde releasers (i.e., quaternium-15, dimethylol dimethyl hydantoin, imidazolidinyl urea, and diazolidinyl urea). Formaldehyde releasers release formaldehyde by hydrolysis in the presence of water. Though, the use of formaldehyde in dermatological products has decreased due to concern about its toxicity, the use of formaldehyde releasers has in fact risen and became a common practice.

Due to the risk of contact dermatitis reactions to preservatives, some cosmetic manufacturers have now switched to packaging which would inhibit the entry of microorganisms.

Contact Urticaria

Development of urticaria immediately (within 5-20 minutes) on application of certain products can be immunologically mediated or nonimmunologic. Benzoic acid, sorbic acid and formaldehyde (all preservatives), alcohols, and cinnamic aldehyde (fragrance) can cause nonimmunologic contact urticaria (NICU). Alcohols, menthol, benzophenones, henna, parabens, polyethylene glycol, polysorbate 60 (emulsifier), and salicylic acid are some of the causes of immunologically mediated CU.

Photoallergic Contact Dermatitis and Phototoxic Contact Dermatitis

Most often caused by fragrances in products (methyl coumarins, musk ambrette), antibacterial agents and sunscreen agents (Para-aminobenzoic acid, benzophenones, dibenzoylmethane).[14,15]

Some ingredients may cause stinging in some individuals and this is reproducible on repeated tests with the same chemical ("light face"). These patients complain of stinging or burning within minutes after applying a product and this intensifies over the next 5-10 minutes after which it resolves, spontaneously.[6] The list of usual culprits is as follows:
- Slight stingers: Benzene, phenol, salicylic acid, and resorcinol
- Moderate: Propylene glycol, dimethyl sulfoxide (DMSO), diethyltoluamide (DEET - mosquito repellent), and benzoyl peroxide
- Severe: Crude coal tar, hydrochloric acid, sodium hydroxide, and phosphoric acid.

PRODUCTS BETTER TOLERATED IN SENSITIVE SKIN

- Inorganic sunscreens: Inorganic sunscreens, which contain microfine preparations of zinc and titanium oxide. These metal oxides are inherently inert and are not absorbed into the skin and are therefore recommended over organic sunscreens in patients with sensitive skin[16]
- Allantoin: It is naturally found in comfrey root but can be synthesized by alkaline oxidation of uric acid in a cool environment[17]
- Green tea extract: Green tea (*Camellia sinensis*) contains polyphenols such as epicatechin and epigallocatechin and is prepared by steaming and drying the fresh tea leaves and carefully avoiding the oxidation of polyphenols. Topically applied green tea extract has been found to reduce ultraviolet B (UVB) induced inflammation in patients of sensitive skin[17]
- Ginkgo biloba: This plant extract contains flavonoids and unique polyphenols such as terpenoids, which have potent anti inflammatory effect. This plant also has an anti-oxidant effect and also, alters the microcirculation of skin at the level of capillary bed and arterioles thereby reducing the erythema[17]
- Aloe vera: This product released from the leaves of plant contains 99.5% water and a complex mixture of mucopolysaccharides, amino acids, hydroxyquinone glycosides and amino acids. The cutaneous effects of aloe vera include decreased bacterial skin colonization, enhanced wound healing, and reduced inflammation.[17]

Chamomile, sunflower oil, bisabolol and white tea extract are also known to be beneficial in sensitive skins.

EXPERIMENTAL AGENTS

Certain chemicals are currently under investigation as agents that could lower skin sensitivity:

- 4-tert-butylcyclohexanol: Vanilloid receptor type-1 (TRPV-1) receptor is involved in the transmission of burning pain and pruritus from skin. The activation of this receptor has been implicated in the pathogenesis of sensitive skin.[1] A 4-tert-butylcyclohexanol has been identified as a potent antagonist of

this receptor. In a study by Kueper et al., it was found that 4-tert-butylcyclohexanol significantly reduced capsaicin mediated TRPV-1 activation, which lead to significant reduction in burning and itching in patients with sensitive skin[18]
- Bacterial lysate: Bifidobacterium longum extract when applied to the skin, significantly reduced burning and itching sensation in patients of sensitive skin[1]
- Thus, exercising some care in the selection of products in individuals with sensitive skin is of utmost importance to avoid further worsening and to ensure compliance.

CONCLUSION

The treatment of sensitive skin thus poses a significant medical challenge which can be overcome by educating the patient regarding the selection of products to be used for his/her skin and following a few basic guidelines which have been outlined in this chapter.

REFERENCES

1. Inamadar AC, Palit A. Sensitive skin: An overview. Indian J Dermatol Venereol Leprol. 2013;79:9-16.
2. Pedro P, Catarina R, Catarina P, et al. Is there any barrier impairment in sensitive skin?: A quantitative analysis of sensitive skin by mathematical modeling of transepidermal water loss desorption curves. Skin Res Technol. 2011;17:181-5.
3. Christensen M, Kligman AM. An improved procedure for conducting lactic acid stinging tests on facial skin. J Sot Cosmet Chem. 1996;47:1-11.
4. Agner T, Serup J. Quantification of the DMSO response: A test for assessment of sensitive skin. Clin Exp Dermatol. 1989;14:214-7.
5. Agner T, Serup J. Skin reactions to irritants assessed by noninvasive bioengineering methods. Contact Dermatitis. 1989;20:352-9.
6. Frosch PJ, Kligman AM. Method for appraising the sting capacity of topically applied substances. J Soc Cosmet Chem. 1977;28:197-209.
7. Muizzuddin N, Marenus KD, Maes DH. Factors defining sensitive skin and its treatment. Am J Contact Dermat. 1998;9(3):170-5.
8. Lev-Tov H, Maibach HI. The Sensitive Skin Syndrome. Indian J Dermatol. 2012;57(6):419-23.
9. Draelos ZD. Sensitive skin: Perceptions, evaluation, and treatment. Contact Dermatitis. 1997;8:67-78
10. Amin S, Maibach HI. Cosmetic intolerance syndrome: Pathophysiology and management. Cosmet Dermatol. 1996;9:34-42.

11. Maibach HI, Engasser PG. Dermatitis due to cosmetics. In: Fisher AA, (Ed). Contact Dermatitis, 3rd ed,. Philadelphia, PA; Lea & Febiger: 1986. pp. 368-93.
12. Draelos ZD. Sensitive skin and contact dermatitis. In: Draelos ZD, editor. Cosmetics and dermatological problems and solutions. 3rd edition. NW; CRC Press; 2011. pp. 27-33
13. Adams RM, Maibach HI. A five-year study of cosmetic reactions. J Am Acad Dermatol. 1985;13:1062-9.
14. Goossens A. Contact-Allergic Reactions to Cosmetics. J Allergy (Cairo). 2011;2011: 467071.
15. De Leo VA, Harber VC. Contact photodermatitis. In: Fisher AA, editor. Contact dermatitis, 3rd edn. Philadelphia; Lea & Febiger: 1986. pp. 454-69.
16. More BD. Physical sunscreens: On the comeback trail. Indian J Dermatol. Venereol Leprol. 2007;73:80-5.
17. Draelos ZD. Treatments for sensitive skin: An update. In: Berardesca E, Fluhr JW, Maibach HI, (Eds). Dermatology: Clinical and Basic Science Series, Sensitive Skin Syndrome, 1st edn. New York: Informa Healthcare; 2006. pp. 245–53.
18. Kueper T, Krohn M, Haustedt LO, et al. Inhibition of TRPV1 for the treatment of sensitive skin. Exp Dermatol. 2010;19:980-6.

CHAPTER 9

Care of Sensitive Skin in Newborns

Indrashis Podder, Rashmi Sarkar

INTRODUCTION

Skin is the largest organ of our body responsible for a myriad of vital functions like maintenance of water and electrolyte homeostasis, thermoregulation, antimicrobial defense (physical and chemical barrier), protection from trauma, radiation, chemicals and toxins, immunomodulation, and synthesis of vitamin; apart from cosmesis.[1] Neonatal skin differs considerably from adult skin, thus mandating special care for its proper functioning. Mothers and caregivers should be made aware about these special measures to ensure healthy and normal skin for their babies. This chapter discusses the major characteristics of neonatal skin, its differences with adult skin, and measures for proper care.

DIFFERENCES BETWEEN NEONATAL SKIN AND ADULT SKIN

Although the neonatal skin bears structural resemblance to adult skin, there are several conspicuous differences pertaining to the physiology, biochemistry, and adnexae (Table 1). As a result of these differences, neonatal skin behaves differently from adult skin in several aspects as tabulated in box 1.

The role of various practices followed in most settings in the care of neonatal skin has been discussed below briefly.

Table 1: Neonatal skin and adult skin—structural differences

Skin structure	Neonatal skin	Adult skin
Epidermis	Thinner cells, fewer layers of stratum corneum, reduced melanin content	Increased thickness of stratum corneum, normal melanin content
Dermo-epidermal junction	Weak (less cohesion)	Strong (more cohesion)
Dermis	Thinner with less elasticity	Thicker and more elastic
Sweat glands	Secretory cells undifferentiated, more dense distribution, less sweating potential	Fully developed sweat glands, distribution less dense, normal sweating capacity
Hair	Lanugo and vellus hair	Vellus and terminal hair
Nerve and vascular system	Not properly developed, unmyelinated nerves	Fully developed and functional
Permeability	Increased absorption due to higher surface area to body weight ratio and increased permeability to fat soluble substances	Less permeability (selective permeability)
Biochemistry	Skin pH <5 (acid mantle); increased free fatty acid content	Skin pH is ~5.5; less free fatty acids

---

BOX 1   **Neonatal skin and adult skin—functional differences**

- Incomplete development of the epidermis leading to altered water-electrolyte homeostasis (increased transepidermal water loss and increased percutaneous absorption) and disturbed thermoregulation
- Increased susceptibility to microbial infections and irritant induced damage due to ill-developed physical barrier (stratum corneum)
- Reduced melanin content making the neonatal skin more vulnerable to ultraviolet light induced damage
- Cautious use of soaps and cleansers is mandated in neonates, as they may further disturb the underdeveloped epidermal barrier and acid mantle, thus leading to dryness and extensive damage
- Reduced chance of colonization by microorganisms because of acidic skin pH in neonates (acid mantle); thus care should be taken to maintain this acid mantle

Role of Vernix Caseosa

Vernix caseosa is a naturally occurring lipid-rich substance covering the newborn babies. It primarily consists of water (81%), lipid (cholesterol, squalene, and wax) and proteins;[2] mostly secreted by the sebaceous glands.[3] The vernix helps immensely in the transition from intrauterine to extrauterine life by preventing loss of fluid and electrolytes/reducing transepidermal water loss (TEWL), thermoregulation, and exerting antioxidant, anti-infective, wound healing, moisturizing, and skin cleansing properties.[4] Traditionally, the vernix has been wiped off neonatal skin; however, in view of its beneficial effects, the World Health Organization has recommended leaving vernix intact on the skin surface after birth, till it sheds off naturally by 6 hours.[4]

Bathing after Birth

The first bath is recommended once the newborn becomes hemodynamically stable and its body temperature is stabilized, usually 2–6 hours after birth in a term infant.[5] However, delayed bathing is advised in winter and/or for low birth weight babies.[1] Clean or sterile lukewarm water (<37°C) should be used for the first birth, not more than 5 minutes, as prolonged bathing may lead to increased dryness.[6] Soaps and cleansers should not be used as they may damage the ill-developed skin barrier. After bathing, the neonate should be dried quickly and thoroughly from head to toe, followed by wrapping in a warm dry towel and placed next to the mother. The first bath is essential to remove vernix and blood from the neonatal skin and also minimize risk of contamination from the maternal blood (human immunodeficiency virus and hepatitis B).

Role of Cleansers and Soaps

Cleansers are chemical substances composed of a surfactant or detergent, intended to remove dirt, sweat, dead skin cells, bacteria, and other debris from the skin surface. Cleansers are of two broad types—alkaline soaps and acidic or neutral synthetic detergents (syndets).[1] Soaps are prepared by saponification, i.e., action of alkali on animal fat or vegetable fat; the latter being replaced by lauryl sulfate or its derivatives in syndets.

The Sensitive Skin: Treatment Modalities and Cosmeceuticals

The major component of cleansers and soaps is surfactant, which acts by decreasing the surface tension between water and air, thus creating a foaming action which allows the fat soluble impurities to be removed from the skin.[6] However, excess use of these surfactants must be avoided to prevent the loss of essential lipids from the neonatal skin.

Minimal use of alkaline cleansers and soaps is recommended in the neonatal period, preferably restricted to the groins, axilla, and diaper areas as they may cause damage to the skin in several ways:[1]

- They may lead to excess absorption of skin lipids, resulting in lipid depleted areas, thus interfering with the barrier function of the skin
- Surfactants may interact with proteins present in the stratum corneum leading to their denaturation, thus further weakening the skin barrier and leading to cutaneous irritation
- The alkaline soaps and cleansers increase the pH of skin, thus nullifying the effect of acid mantle, leading to increased microbial colonization and TEWL, resulting in increased incidence of infections, dryness, and roughness.

The authors recommend the use of syndets and other soap substitutes (nonsoap surfactants and lipid free lotions) mostly in flexures as these substances have a pH closer to the normal skin, thus being less irritant and harmful than conventional soaps. Another distinct advantage of these nonsoap substances is that they do not alter the "acid-mantle" of neonatal skin, thus the cutaneous microbiome remains unaltered.[7]

Nonsoap lipid free lotions usually contain a syndet (surfactant) and emollients like glycerin, cetyl alcohol, and propylene glycol, but no oils or fat. These liquid products can clean without water. They can be safely applied to the dry skin, rubbed to produce lather, and wiped off with a soft cloth.[1]

However, a major disadvantage of these soap-substitutes is their high cost and rapid rate of degeneration. Cocoyl isethionate, sodium lauryl sulfate, and betaines are some of the commonly used soap substitutes.

Additionally, all these substances must be physically and chemically stable, devoid of fragrance and colors, and contain an emollient to avoid irritation.[1] However, minimal use of these chemical substances is advised in the neonatal period.

ROLE OF BABY POWDERS

Baby powders are extensively used in the Indian scenario aimed at absorbing moisture during the hot and humid weather to keep the intertriginous areas dry. However, excessive use of these powders may lead to blockade of the sweat apparatus leading to miliaria.[8] Accidental inhalation and contact dermatitis are other potential hazards. Thus, the authors recommend avoidance of baby powders during the neonatal period as their risks outweigh the gains. However, recently liquid baby powders are being marketed. These are non-talc liquid lotions which transform into a silky, protective stay-dry powder to keep the skin cool and dry (e.g., Huggies® liquid baby powder, Johnson's® liquid talc, Carter's® liquid baby powder, etc.). They contain natural and certified organic oils being safe for the neonatal skin. They have the advantage of being less messy with minimum risk of inhalation and contact dermatitis. However, long-term use and further research are required before they can be safely recommended.

Role of Emollients and Moisturizers

Emollients/moisturizers are natural or synthetic chemical substances primarily containing lipids which help to keep the skin soft and supple. They may be naturally derived (containing animal/vegetable derived lipids or mineral oils) or synthetic in nature. Emollients can be broadly grouped under the following heads:
- Hydrocarbons—vaseline, paraffin
- Fatty substance—cetyl/stearyl alcohol
- Waxes—bees wax, lanolin
- Oils—mineral oils, vegetable oils like coconut oil, palm kernel oil, ground nut oil, olive oil, and mustard oil.

Based on the type of formulation/vehicle used, emollients/moisturizers can be further categorized into two types:
1. Creams—major vehicle in water (oil-in-water emulsion); less sticky and less occlusive, thus being more preferred in the hot, humid Indian weather
2. Ointment—major vehicle in oil (water-in-oil emulsion); more sticky and more occlusive.

In the Indian setup, vegetable oils are used most frequently because of their considerable efficacy, low side effect profile and bearable cost, thus called "poor man's moisturizer." About 95% of each vegetable oil is composed primarily of triglycerides with meager amounts of mono and diglycerides. Coconut oil and palm oil contains mainly saturated fatty acids while other oils largely contain unsaturated fatty acids (oleic acid, linoleic acid, and linolenic acid). Among these oils, coconut oil has been found to be most effective.[9] Contrary to the popular belief, mustard oil happens to be inferior to coconut oil, as it may occasionally lead to contact dermatitis; although incidence is very low in India.[9,10] The widely popular olive oil is also inferior to sunflower oil and safflower oil in this regard.[9] Argan oil, a recent introduction, has also been found to be effective having additional antioxidant properties.[9]

Application of emollients and moisturizers to the neonatal skin serves several functions as listed below:
- Reduces neonatal peeling and scaling effectively without any notable adverse effect
- Maintains barrier function, thus keeping the skin soft and supple diminishing the chance of atopic dermatitis
- Reduces irritation in the napkin area, thus reducing chances of diaper dermatitis.

Role of Massage

Proper massaging technique should be employed while applying these emollients to derive maximal benefits. Darmstadt et al.[11] have shown that lubricant oil massage is more effective than dry massage. Moderate pressure massage with passive movement (flexion and extension) of the limbs has been shown to provide the optimum benefit. Overzealous and vigorous massage should be avoided as it may lead to physical injuries and enhance the chance of infection. Some of the important beneficial effects of proper massaging include weight gain, better sleep-wake cycle, enhanced neuromotor development, emotional bonding, and lower rates of nosocomial infections in both term and preterm babies.[9]

CARE OF SPECIFIC AREAS

Although the whole skin has to be taken care of, some specific areas require additional care like the diaper area and scalp as discussed below.

Care of the Diaper Area[1]

The diaper area is a large moist, humid, and occluded environment where the skin remains in contact with strong alkaline substances like urine and feces thereby increasing the chances of maceration and microbial infections. The basic pathology is skin barrier dysfunction due to these caustic substances.

Mothers must be instructed to change diapers frequently air-drying the skin in between. Emollients/moisturizers or vegetable oils may be applied at regular intervals to keep the barrier function intact. Zinc oxide containing emollients are preferred to the bland alternatives if diaper dermatitis develops. If feces is present, it should be gently wiped off (front to back) using soft cotton wool soaked in warm water. Soap-free baby lotions/syndets may be used to clean the areas if the feces are adherent. The diapers should be regularly washed in lukewarm water followed by rinsing and drying.

Care of the Scalp

Infantile seborrheic dermatitis may affect neonatal scalp (cradle cap) as well as the other body folds and seborrhoeic areas; with maximum occurrence reported in the first 3 months (71.7%).[12] It is usually self-limiting, clearing by 4-6 months in most cases.[13] However, this is a concern to parents and they often seek medical intervention. Baby shampoos may be used to remove the crusts and scales. Topical ketoconazole and zinc pyrithione lotions may be used safely with minimum contact period as negligible systemic absorption has been reported.[12] Anti-inflammatory agents like topical hydrocortisone cream have also been recommended in severe cases, although concerns have been raised about their side-effects.[14] Historically, biotin has also been postulated as a treatment, because similar scalp lesions to seborrheic dermatitis are seen as part of biotinidase deficiency conditions.[12] Recently, some complementary and alternative medicines are also being used as treatment like licochalcone (extracted from *Glycyrrhiza inflata*).[15] Several authors recommend application of mineral or vegetable oils (e.g., olive oil) to soften scales and lift scales, followed by brushing to mechanically remove scales;[1,12] but this view is debatable as it promotes a favorable environment for the yeast *Malassezia furfur* to proliferate and may theoretically worsen the condition.[12] Concerns have been raised regarding the use of keratolytics (salicylic acid) and selenium sulfide shampoos in neonates because of the risk of systemic absorption and scalp discoloration.[12] Baby shampoos contain both cleansers and lather enhancers, the later necessary for psychological effects rather than cleaning;[16] apart from minimal amount of preservatives, dyes, antioxidants, chelators, and conditioners. These shampoos should be ideally free from fragrance and other anti-inflammatory agents to avoid contact dermatitis. An ideal baby shampoo should have its pH close to that of tears (around 7) in order to be nonirritating to the baby's eyes (e.g., Cetaphil® baby shampoo, Johnson's® baby shampoo, etc.).

CONCLUSION

The neonatal skin is extremely delicate and sensitive, so proper care must be taken to keep it healthy. First bath should be given about 4-6 hours post birth with clean, lukewarm water. The authors recommend minimum usage of soaps, cleansers, and shampoos. In case of need, neutral or slightly acidic pH syndets (synthetic detergents) and soap-free lotions may be used especially in the groins, axilla, and diaper area. Emollients may be properly massaged to keep the skin soft and supple, coconut oil being a cost effective option. However, limited usage is recommended in hot and humid climate. Baby powders are better avoided as they have a skewed risk-benefit ratio although recently introduced nontalc, liquid baby powders may be used safely.

REFERENCES

1. Sarkar R, Basu S, Agrawal RK, et al. Skin care for the newborn. Indian pediatrics. 2010;47:593-8.
2. Hoeger PH, Schreiner V, Klaassen IA, et al. Epidermal barrier lipids in human vernix caseosa: corresponding ceramide pattern in vernix and fetal skin. Br J Dermatol. 2002;146:194-201.
3. Hoath SB, Pickens WL, Visscher MO. The biology of vernix caseosa. Int J Cosmet Sci. 2006;28(5):319-33.
4. Singh G, Archana G. Unraveling the mystery of vernix caseosa. Indian J Dermatol. 2008;53(2):54.
5. Basu S, Gupta P. Care of the normal newborn. In: Gupta P, editor. Essential pediatric Nursing. New Delhi: CBS Publishers and Distributors; 2007. p. 217-26.

6. Dhar S. Newborn skin care revisited. Indian J Dermatol. 2007;52:1.
7. Hugill K. Neonatal skin cleansing revisited: Whether or not to use skin cleansing products. Br J Midwifery. 2014;22:694-98.
8. Mofenson HC, Greensher J, DiTomasso A, et al. Baby Powder—A Hazard! Pediatrics. 1981;68:265-6.
9. Sarkar R, Podder I, Gokhale N, et al. Use of vegetable oils in dermatology: An overview. Int J Dermatol. 2017;56(11):1080-86.
10. Pasricha JS, Gupta R, Gupta SK. Contact hypersensitivity to mustard khal and mustard oil. Indian J Dermatol Venereol Leprol. 1975;51:108-10.
11. Darmstadt GL, Mao-Qiang M, Chi E, et al. Impact of topical oils on the skin barrier: Possible implications for neonatal health in developing countries. Acta Paediatr. 2002;91:546-54.
12. Victoire A, Magin P, Coughlan J, et al. Interventions for infantile seborrhoeic dermatitis (including cradle cap). The Cochrane Library. 2014.
13. Gelmetti C, Grimalt R. Infantile seborrhoeic dermatitis. In: Irvine A, Hoeger P, Yan A, editor(s). Harper's textbook of pediatric dermatology. West Sussex, UK: Wiley-Blackwell; 2011. pp. 35.1-35.
14. Arora V, Arora S. Management of infantile seborrheic dermatitis. Am Fam Physician. 2007;75(6):807.
15. Wananukul S, Chatproedprai S, Charutragulchai W. Randomized, double-blind, split-side comparison study of moisturizer containing licochalcone vs 1% hydrocortisone in the treatment of infantile seborrhoeic dermatitis. J Eur Acad Dermatol Venereol. 2012;26(7):894-7.
16. D'Souza P, Rathi SK. Shampoo and conditioners: What a dermatologist should know? Indian J Dermatol. 2015;60:248.

10
CHAPTER

Skin Care of Aged Skin

Indrashis Podder, Rashmi Sarkar

INTRODUCTION

Aging is an inevitable physiological process associated with several anatomical, physical, and psychosocial changes. With improvement in the world of medicine, more old people are alive today than have ever been in the past. According to the World Health Organization (WHO) definition, people above 60 years of age belong to the elderly/geriatric age group.[1] The World's population is growing and aging; it is estimated that the world will host 1.2 billion people aged 60 by 2025, which would rise to 1.9 billion by 2050.[2] The Indian demography is also showing a similar trend with its elderly population expected to increase dramatically over the next few decades.

The aging process takes its toll on the skin also leading to several conspicuous skin changes in this population like compromised barrier function and mechanical protection, delayed wound healing and immune responses, and altered thermoregulation with reduced secretion of sweat and sebum. On the cellular level, the content of natural moisturizing factors and lipids is reduced in the stratum corneum, resulting in decreased lamellar bilayers and poorer water-holding capacity. Additionally, chronic diseases, drugs, and environmental factors including detrimental skin care habits increase the risk of skin damage.[3]

CLASSIFICATION OF CUTANEOUS AGING

Cutaneous aging can be broadly grouped under two heads depending on the pathophysiology:

1. Intrinsic aging—inevitable change attributable to the passage of time also called true aging; genetically determined physiological phenomenon
2. Extrinsic aging—occurs due to superposition of changes on intrinsic aging attributable to chronic sun exposure (photoaging), other environmental factors (pollution, toxins, etc.) and some internal factors like altered hormonal milieu induced by senile changes in organs.

EFFECTS OF CUTANEOUS AGING

The age-related skin changes often result in different types of skin disorders and skin injuries. The most common dermatological problem in the elderly is dryness/xerosis also called xerosis cutis, with prevalence ranging from 30–85%.[3-5] This occurs due to depletion of water and natural moisturizing factors in the elderly skin. Dryness of skin subsequently leads to generalized pruritus, which severely worsens the quality of life and status of skin.[6]

The elderly patients are also at risk of skin injuries like skin tears or other partial to full-thickness wounds such as superficial pressure ulcers; their prevalence ranging from 2–40%.[3,7] Flattened dermoepidermal junction and increased skin stiffness increases the risk of such skin injuries in this population.[3]

Another common cutaneous problem in the geriatric age group is incontinence-associated dermatoses. Excessive moisture from urine and/or stools leads to over hydration and chemical irritation of the epidermis while physical insult (e.g., cleansing) destroys the epidermis and dermis. Incontinence-associated dermatoses affect almost 50% of all geriatric patients at some point of time.[8]

SKIN CARE IN THE ELDERLY

Adequate skin care is of paramount importance to maintain skin barrier, integrity, and optimum skin health, especially in high-risk populations like the geriatric age group. However, there is lack of specific guidelines in this regard in the present set up. So, the authors have tried to elaborate the optimum skin care measures, in the elderly in this chapter.

The Sensitive Skin: Treatment Modalities and Cosmeceuticals

Geriatric skin care may be broadly discussed under two heads:
1. Care of dry skin
2. Prevention of skin injuries.

Care of Dry Skin

Use of syndet bars during bathing and subsequent use of moisturizers/emollients has been shown to reduce skin dryness.[9] Excessive bathing has been found to exacerbate skin dryness, so short duration of baths is recommended.[3]

Application of creams and lotions containing humectants like urea, lactic acid, and glycerin have been found to reduce skin dryness by decreasing the transepidermal water loss (TEWL), thus maintaining the skin hydration. Application of dimethicone-containing skin products also retards TEWL, thus keeping the skin supple. Humectant containing preparations have been found to be more efficacious than bland preparations.[3] However, no significant difference has been observed in the efficacy of different humectants.[10] Recently, a chitin-glucan containing cream has been introduced, which has been shown to improve skin hydration in comparison to placebo.[11]

Emollients and moisturizers also protect the skin from chemical injuries resulting from incontinence associated dermatoses by maintaining the integrity of skin barrier.

Based on evidence obtained from systemic reviews, combining emollients with humectants seems to be the best strategy to manage skin dryness.

Prevention of Skin Injuries

Injuries may damage the skin integrity, thus affecting its water retaining capacity, aggravating dryness and different pathologies. Use of special soaps and nondetergent cleansers, with or without moisturizers, has been found to protect the skin from different types of injuries like tears and abrasions. Combination of emollients and humectants exert an additional protective effect by restoring the skin barrier function.

CONCLUSION

Proper measures should be undertaken to take care of the skin in the elderly population as it is a challenging situation for the treating physician and is becoming more important with each passing day. Prevention of skin injuries and maintenance of skin hydration are the common objectives to attain this goal. The authors have mentioned several modalities to take proper care of the skin in this vulnerable population. However, more trials are needed to search for better agents to address the growing needs of the geriatric population.

REFERENCES

1. Ibrahim NK, Ghabrah TM, Qadi M. Morbidity profile of elderly attended/admitted in Jeddah health facilities, Saudi Arabia. Bull High Inst Public Health. 2005;35:173-90.
2. McMurdo ME. A healthy old age: Realistic or futile goal? BMJ. 2000;321(7269): 1149-51.
3. Kottner J, Lichterfeld A, Blume-Peytavi U. Maintaining skin integrity in the aged: A systematic review. Brit J Dermatol. 2013;169(3):528-42.
4. Paul C, Maumus-Robert S, Mazereeuw-Hautier J, et al. Prevalence and risk factors for xerosis in the elderly: A cross-sectional epidemiological study in primary care. Dermatology. 2011;223:260-5.
5. Hahnel E, Lichterfeld A, Blume-Peytavi U, et al. The epidemiology of skin conditions in the aged: A systematic review. J Tissue Viability. 2017;26(1):20-8.
6. Valdes-Rodriguez R, Stull C, Yosipovitch G. Chronic pruritus in the elderly: Pathophysiology, diagnosis and management. Drugs Aging. 2015;32(3):201-15.
7. LeBlanc K, Baranoski S. Skin tears: State of the science: Consensus statements for the prevention, prediction, assessment, and treatment of skin tears. Adv Skin Wound Care. 2011;24:2-15.
8. Gray M. Optimal management of incontinence-associated dermatitis in the elderly. Am J Clin Dermatol. 2010;11:201-10.
9. Hardy MA. What can you do about your patient's dry skin? J Gerontol Nurs. 1996;22: 10-8.
10. Sch€olermann A, Bohnsack K, Stephan K, et al. Efficacy and safety of Eucerin 10% Urea cream in xerotic aged skin. Z Hautkr. 1999;10:557-62.
11. Quatresooz P, Pierard-Franchimont C, Szepetiuk G, et al. Fungal chitin–glucan scaffold for managing diabetic xerosis of the feet in menopausal women. Expert Opin Pharmacother. 2009;10:2221-9.

11
CHAPTER

Cosmetics for Sensitive Skin: Practical Tips

Minal Patwardhan, Akreti S Sobti

INTRODUCTION

The term "sensitive skin" is used to describe skin which easily breaks out in rashes, get blotchy and itchy, or develops stinging sensation in response to various factors, which may be physical (ultraviolet radiation, heat, cold, and wind), chemical (cosmetics, soap, water, and pollution), psychological (stress), or hormonal (menstrual cycle).[1,2]

The skin reacts with onset of erythema and/or prickling, burning, or tingling sensations. It is commonly a self-diagnosed condition and is typically unaccompanied by any obvious physical signs of irritation when the patient actually presents to the doctor.[3]

Increasing social media advertising, lifestyle changes, and easy accessibility to a variety of cosmetics and cosmetic procedures has in reality increased this "sensitive skin" phenomenon. More and more people are indiscriminately using new products purely because of hyped up advertising and especially celebrities recommending a wide variety of them!

Dermatologists' opinion dictates that a problem-free skin is best not tampered with and experimentation with various products is truly unnecessary. Sensitive skin has been variously classified into distinct subgroups of clinical sensitivities; the two most often quoted are by Pons-Guiraud and Muizzuddin, respectively (Table 1).[4,5]

KNOWING YOUR SKIN TYPE[6]

The main aspect of forming a skin care routine is finding the right product that suits one's skin type. So the question arises as to "how

Cosmetics for Sensitive Skin: Practical Tips

Table 1: Classifications of sensitive skin

Classification	Features	Subgroups
Pons-Guiraud	Very sensitive	Reactive to various exogenous and endogenous stimuli with acute and chronic symptoms
	Environmentally sensitive	Clear dry thin skin with tendency to blush or flush with environmental trigger
	Cosmetically sensitive	Skin that reacts to a specific and definable cosmetic product
Muizzuddin	Delicate skin	Characterized by easily disrupted barrier function not accompanied by a rapid or intense inflammatory response
	Reactive skin	Characterized by a strong inflammatory response without a significant increase in permeability
	Stingers	Skin heightened neurosensory perception to minor cutaneous stimulation

does one determine one's skin type?" However, before we determine skin type, one has to outline the factors influencing the skin type. There are both external and internal factors as listed below.

Internal Factors

- Hormones
- Skin disorders
- Genetic predisposition
- Diet
- Stress.

External Factors

- Smoking and passive smoking
- Medication
- Prolong sun exposure/no sunscreen application
- Climate
- Pollution

The Sensitive Skin: Treatment Modalities and Cosmeceuticals

- Skin care routine/products used
- Alcohol.

SKIN TYPE DETERMINATION

The five main conventional variants of skin types are dry, oily, normal, combination, and sensitive skin, extrapolated from the first classification given by Helena Rubinstein in 1910. Each of them can be determined by their behavior after application of a basic and bland moisturizer. It has to be kept in mind that anyone can have multiple skin types during their lifetime, depending on the trigger factors as discussed above.

To begin the process of determination, one has to clean the face with a gentle cleanser and apply a bland emollient/moisturizer over face and check the face after 2 hours. The interpretation is given in table 2.

CHOOSING THE RIGHT PRODUCT FOR YOUR SKIN[6]

Once the skin type has been determined, the next step is to understand what kind of skin product can be applied over the face. The composition of the product is the same, however, the base texture differs for different skin types. Given below is a table indicating what kind of product would suit which kind of skin type (Table 3).

Recently, Baumann has introduced four basic parameters in the Baumann Skin Type Indicator that more accurately characterize skin types.[7] By evaluating skin according to these parameters—dry or oily, sensitive or resistant, pigmented or non-pigmented, and

Table 2: Skin type determination

Skin behavior	Type of skin
Some areas (T zone) oily and some area (cheeks) dry	Combination skin
Most areas appear dry and scaly and feel tightness	Dry skin
Feels oily and sticky	Oily skin
Feels no change (not oily/dry)	Normal skin
Looks red and patchy, feels tight and irritated	Sensitive skin

Table 3: **Choosing the right product for your skin type**

Product texture	Skin type			
	Oily	Combination	Dry	Normal
Lotion		•	•	•
Cream			•	•
Gel	•	•		•
Serum	•	•	•	•
Liquid	•	•		•
Powder	•			

wrinkled or unwrinkled—and thus differentiating among the 16 permutations of possible skin types, patients and dermatologists can more easily identify the most suitable topical treatments. He divided sensitive skin (S) patients into four types: acne, rosacea, burning/stinging, and allergic, each of which would require different cosmetic products and skin care products.[7]

Daily Skin Care Routine

Healthy skin can be achieved with well formulated skin products and avoiding excessive sun exposure (with physical or chemical sunscreen). One can obtain the best possible skin for one's skin type and age. Serious investigation over the years has now proved how antioxidants, anti-irritants, and skin repairing ingredients are important to heal sensitive skin.

How does One Realistically Deal with Sensitive Skin?

We need to understand that every skin type is individualistic. There is no standard regimen for skin care because very few people would have a constant skin type. It varies from time-to-time as mentioned earlier.

The "hypoallergenic" claim of many cosmetics is actually meaningless because it is not a guarantee of a gentle or safer formula as there are no accepted standardized testing methods of any kind to determine whether a product qualifies as hypoallergenic.

Conversely, there is no law that prevents a company from labeling their product hypoallergenic!

The ingredient alcohol is to be watched out for in products. Look for "specially denatured alcohol followed by a number" in ingredient list. This causes dryness, free radical damage, and impairs skin healing.

High amounts of fragrance in products whether synthetic or "natural" can cause chronic irritation and damage skin collagen and lead to a worsening of sensitive skin. Lavender oil, specifically lindool, can be cytotoxic on topical application. Lavender leaves contain camphor which is a known skin irritant.

Daily Regimen

There are three basic skin care facts:
1. Any and every skin care routine must include sunscreen
2. One must follow the skin care routine consistently
3. A trial and error phase is needed to achieve the final skin care routine that suits each individual.

The routine should include:
- Cleanser: A gentle water soluble cleanser helps remove debris, oil, and also helps the skin to remain healthy. It is actually best to use liquid preparations as opposed to bar soaps because they can cause clogging of pores
- Toner: Using a toner daily has its own risk and benefits. A well formulated toner can smoothen and calm the skin. Toner with skin repairing ingredients hydrates the skin surface. Toners containing alcohol are best avoided
- Moisturizer: All skin types benefit from a moisturizer. Depending on the skin type either a cream, lotion, or gel-based moisturizer can be used. It replaces the dull, dry patches over the skin
- Sunscreen: This is the part of the daily regimen that is the most essential of all. It helps in protecting our skin from sun damage
- Scrubbing does not extract blackheads; in fact scrubbing daily strips your skin of its protective layers exposing the living cells to the environment leading to worsening of sensitivity. Exfoliation is best done using alpha-hydroxy acids (AHA) or beta-hydroxy acid (BHA) products and masks at suitable intervals, they hydrate and exfoliate simultaneously.

INSTRUCTIONS FOR COSMETIC AND MAKEUP USE FOR SENSITIVE SKIN

Makeup is a personal choice and what matters most are the texture, application, and performance. Essentials of makeup usage in sensitive skins are to avoid very heavy makeup and particularly concealers. These increase clogging and removal is difficult causing skin sensitivity. Sensitive skin types would do well to use a primer or a moisturizer especially containing bisabolol prior to applying makeup. This will protect the skin and also facilitate makeup removal.

Use a gentle cleanser first to remove makeup and then follow it up with a makeup remover that can be brand specific or a gentle soothing milk or micellar water. Eye makeup specially requires gentle removers. Check the expiry of your makeup especially creams, lotions, mascara, and lipsticks, which last for 6 months to a year. Nail lacquer even though distant can cause skin sensitivity due to contact. Strictly avoid alcohol based topical applications.

Following are some other salient points to keep in mind:
- Powdered cosmetics are preferred over the other forms
- Eyeliners and mascara should be of black color
- Avoid using nail polish
- Use cosmetics with lesser number of ingredients (preferably <10)
- Fresh cosmetics should be used always and they should be removable with water
- Lighter tone of colors should be used for eye shadow.

CONCLUSION

Choosing the right product is actually by trial and error for any individual; but certain salient tips can be kept in mind while prescribing to make the process smoother and avoid causing further sensitivity by known culprits.

REFERENCES

1. Inamadar AC, Palit A. Sensitive skin: An overview. Indian J Dermatol Venereol Leprol. 2013;79:9-16.
2. Willis CM, Shaw S, Lacharriere OD, et al. Sensitive skin: An epidemiological study. Br J Dermatol. 2001;145:258-63.

3. Loffler H, Aramaki J, Effendy I, et al. Sensitive skin. In: Zhai H, Maibach H, editors. Dermatotoxicology. New York: CRC Press; 2004. p. 123-35.
4. Pons-Guiraud A. Sensitive skin: A complex and Multifactorial syndrome. J Cosmet Dermatol. 2005;3:145-8.
5. Muizzuddin N, Marenus KD, Maes DH. Factors defining sensitive skin and its treatment. Am J Contact Dermat. 1998;9:170-5.
6. Begoun P. Don't go to the cosmetic counter without me, 9th edn. October 2012; pp. 22-3.
7. Baumann L. Understanding and treating various skin types: The Baumann skin type indicator. Dermatol Clin. 2008;26(3):359-73.

12
CHAPTER

Dermatological Procedures in Sensitive Skin

Azin Ayatollahi, Alireza Firooz

INTRODUCTION

Nowadays request for cosmetic and rejuvenation procedures are exceptionally high, and among these patients the number of subjects with sensitive skin is noticeable. To this day, effects of cosmetic and rejuvenation procedures on subjects with sensitive skin have not been studied thoroughly. This chapter endeavors to explore whether popular cosmetic and rejuvenation procedures are suitable and safe for patients with sensitive skin.

SENSITIVE SKIN AND PROCEDURES

A person's skin is said to be sensitive when the skin has subjective hyperreactivity in response to environmental factors and conditions. It is common for those with sensitive skin to report excessive reactions in response to application of sunscreens, cosmetics, and soaps to the skin. Exposure to cold and dry climate is often reported to exacerbate these reactions.[1,2]

A sensitive skin may have a thinner stratum corneum with a reduced corneocyte area resulting in a higher transcutaneous penetration of water-soluble chemicals.[3] An imbalance of intercellular lipid of stratum corneum has already been reported as one factor causing declined barrier function in sensitive skin.[4] Other factors such as changes in the nervous system and/or the structure of the epidermis may also contribute to the declined barrier function in sensitive skin.[5]

The Sensitive Skin: Treatment Modalities and Cosmeceuticals

Among various skin sites on one's body, facial skin has a thinner barrier and a greater density of nerve endings. Further, facial skin is subject to many applications of various cosmetic products, particularly by women. These have led to the conclusion that facial skin is the most common site of skin sensitivity.[6] Within the facial area, the nasolabial fold was reported to be the most sensitive region, followed by the malar eminence, chin, forehead, and upper lip.[7,8]

Most of the dermatological procedures for skin rejuvenation are carried out on the facial region. It should be noted that when such procedures are performed on subjects with sensitive skin, dermatologists should exercise a higher degree of care and attention since, as discussed above, in subjects with sensitive skin, facial skin is the most common site of sensitivity. Skin chemical peels, resurfacing techniques like microdermabrasion or microablation, lasers including ablative and nonablative systems and also hair removal lasers, radiofrequency technologies, botulinum toxins, and soft tissue augmentation are amongst the most common rejuvenation procedures.

Chemical Peeling

In chemical peeling, a chemical solution such as alpha-hydroxy acid, trichloroacetic acid, or phenolic compound is applied to the skin.[9] Depending upon the type and concentration of chemical agent used, the depth of peeling will be different. The chemical agent destroys the upper layers of the skin in a controlled fashion. Accordingly, patients with sensitive skin or those with history of atopic dermatitis are at risk of complications if exposed to chemical peels that go too deep. They are also more prone to develop side effects such as skin irritation and prolonged erythema after chemical peeling. Hence, it is safer to use mild superficial peels in these individuals.

The latest American Society for Dermatosurgery guidelines task force consensus recommendations concluded that there is insufficient evidence to justify delaying treatment with superficial chemical peels in patients on/exposed to isotretinoin within the past 6 months. Data on medium and deep chemical peels was insufficient to make recommendations.

However, in patients with sensitive skin, it would be better to stick to the earlier guidelines and avoid even superficial peels while on/within 6 months after isotretinoin intake.

Microdermabrasion

Microdermabrasion is a noninvasive skin resurfacing technique with noticeable patient satisfaction and mild adverse effects. In contrast to the chemical peeling, performing microdermabrasion does not necessarily need to be avoided on patients with sensitive skin. However, this procedure, which has become very popular for superficial resurfacing, should be carried out with caution.

Most microdermabrasion units are closed-loop, negative-pressure systems which pass aluminum oxide crystals onto the skin, while simultaneously vacuuming the used crystals. Other systems utilize sodium chloride (NaCl) and positive pressure for superficial skin resurfacing.

A study by Rajan et al. demonstrated a statistically significant increase in transepidermal water loss (TEWL), 24 hours after conducting the microdermabrasion (using negative pressure system on one half of the face and positive pressure system on the other half). This may be an evidence that microdermabrasion disrupts the lipid barrier of the epidermis, i.e., a declined barrier function. As a result of this declined barrier function, those with sensitive skin may have more discomfort than those with normal skin during the first few hours after the microdermabrasion procedures. Accordingly, microdermabrasion should be carried out with caution in subjects with sensitive skin and be followed with more rigorous postoperation care. Rajan et al. showed that 7 days after microdermabrasion, there was a drop in TEWL to mean values slightly less than those seen at baseline. This suggests that restoration of barrier function has occurred, with a trend toward improvement in the lipid barrier function over baseline.[10] This finding has been confirmed in other studies too.[11]

Fractional Resurfacing Lasers

Traditional laser resurfacing [ultra-pulsed CO_2 or neodymium-doped:yttrium:aluminum-garnet (Nd:YAG) laser] ablates 100% of the epidermal surface. Fractional ablative lasers deliver microscopic columns of energy for vaporizing myriads of tiny holes covering only a small to moderate percentage of the skin surface. Aforementioned lasers have fewer side effects such as immediate post-treatment erythema, prolonged erythema and heat-induced recall phenomenon.[12] Immediate post-treatment erythema usually resolves within 3–4 days. Prolonged erythema is defined as post-treatment erythema that persists longer than 4 days with nonablative resurfacing and beyond 1 month with ablative treatment.[12] Patients with sensitive skin are more prone to these side effects, and the post laser induced erythema may be more prolonged than the normal skin patients.

Heat-induced recall phenomenon has been observed after skin resurfacing with fractional lasers. After resolution of transient post-treatment wheal-like erythema, some patients experience reappearance of erythematous patches after a hot shower or prolonged exposure to direct sunlight, resulting in a "recall" phenomenon. It appears that there is an activation of neurogenic or histamine- or mast cell-dependent mechanisms responsible for high levels of molecules that produce erythema in the skin.[12] In subjects with sensitive skin due to the changes that occur in their nervous system, the rate of heat induced recall phenomenon might be higher than normal. Thus, we recommend avoiding the use of conventional ablative lasers and being careful in fractional resurfacing lasers for sensitive skin patients.

Hair Removal Lasers

Laser assisted hair removal is one of the most common procedures that has lots of applicants nowadays. It is the treatment of choice for reducing the unwanted hair. Different lasers and light sources are currently available for photoepilation. These lasers operate in the red or near-infrared wavelengths. Ruby laser (694 nm), alexandrite laser (755 nm), diode laser (800–810 nm), Nd:YAG laser (1,064 nm), and intense pulsed light (IPL) (590–1,200 nm) are some examples of aforesaid lasers and light sources.[13,14]

Bouzari et al. showed that the 755-nm alexandrite and the 800 nm diode laser have approximately equal efficacy while the Nd:YAG laser is the least efficacious. Even though the objective of laser-assisted hair removal is to permanently damage follicles, a risk of epidermal injury during the hair removal process does exist.[15]

Methods for protecting the epidermis during laser-assisted hair removal may include contact cooling laser tips and topical application of cooling gels and cryogens. Epidermal cooling serves to reduce the amount of superficial thermal damage sustained upon laser impact. Although various strategies such as cooling systems have been developed, laser procedures still present a risk of adverse effects due to overheating of skin. The most common side effects of laser treatment are erythema and perifollicular edema.[16]

Absorption of laser light by epidermal melanin generates heat. This generated heat is a major contributor in inducing transient erythema. However, transient erythema is not considered as an adverse event. Transient erythema happens by vasodilation, caused by prostaglandin release and direct thermal damage of vessel as a result of the thermal heat generated by laser-skin interaction. Erythema normally clears within several hours with adequate cooling, but it has been reported to last as long as 7 days.[16] Ilknur et al. revealed statistically significant increase in erythema index in the second week in the laser-treated area compared to the control area, which shows that the erythema response with the diode laser can continue up to the second week.[17]

In subjects with sensitive skin, the epidermal cooling during the hair removal procedure may increase skin sensitivity, and the erythema that occurred after treatment may last longer than usual. So physicians should explain to patients with sensitive skin that post laser erythema may be more severe and long lasting.

Botulinum Toxins

One method for treating wrinkles and skin rejuvenation is injection of botulinum toxins. In addition to its rejuvenation properties, botulinum toxin type A has been shown to be effective in prophylactically treating chronic migraines. Botulinum toxin type A's mechanisms for treating chronic migraines, such as a direct effect of neurotoxins on sensory neurons, may have some role in decreasing sensitivity in patient with sensitive skin.[18]

One method that botulinum toxin type A may affect sensory neurons is through inhibiting neuropeptide and neurotransmitter release from peripheral terminals of afferent neurons. Botulinum toxin type A can inhibit a number of neurochemicals released from sensory neurons known to stimulate peripheral nociceptors, including glutamate, substance P, and calcitonin gene-related peptide (CGRP). By reducing the release of these neurochemicals, peripheral sensitization may be reduced. This in turn may indirectly reduce central sensitization.[18]

One other potential antinociceptive effect of botulinum toxin is reducing the expression of transient receptor potential, vanilloid family 1 (TRPV1) in a number of cells and tissues, which can potentially reduce peripheral sensitization. TRPV1 is an ion channel found on some sensory neurons. It is activated by capsaicin, protons, and noxious heat, and is upregulated in tissues during chronic pain and inflammation.[18] TRPV1 activation results in pain or pruritus with a burning component.[5]

In sensitive skin, neurogenic inflammation may result from the release of neurotransmitters such as substance P, calcitonin gene-related peptide and vasoactive intestinal peptide. Release of such neurotransmitters may induce vasodilatation and mast cell degranulation. TRPV1 is also dramatically upregulated by said inflammatory mediators.[5]

To conclude, the authors hypothesized that the same mechanism followed by botulinum toxin type A in treating chronic migraines, may reduce sensitivity in patients with sensitive skin.

Soft Tissue Fillers

Currently available injectable soft tissue fillers such as hyaluronic acid, calcium hydroxylapatite, poly-L-lactic acid, polymethyl methacrylate, and autologous fat have changed the prospect of skin rejuvenation. Among mentioned fillers, hyaluronic acid gel has been mainly used to treat folds and wrinkles associated with facial aging. In general, hyaluronic acid fillers are effective and safe. Side-effects are generally limited to bruising and edema. After injection, patients are advised to apply ice pack to the injected area for up to 10 minutes in every hour. In the next day after injection, additional edema as a result of hydration is expected. This may result in a feeling of soreness, relievable with acetaminophen. Bruising can occur up to 72 hours after injection.[19]

It should be noted that in sensitive skin patients, injection of fillers such as hyaluronic acid may not increase skin sensitivity by itself. However, it is the use of ice packs that may cause increased sensitivity.

CONCLUSION

Among aesthetic procedures discussed in this chapter, carrying out chemical peeling should be avoided in patients with sensitive skin. On the other hand, injecting botulinum toxin, with regard to its effects on sensory neurons, as discussed above, may reduce sensitivity in patients with sensitive skin. Further studies to prove this hypothesis is beneficial. As a final note, since the body of research and studies on the effects of cosmetic and rejuvenation procedures on subjects with sensitive skin are rather thin, more studies in this group of patients are recommended.

REFERENCES

1. Yokota T, Matsumoto M, Sakamaki T, et al. Classification of sensitive skin and development of a treatment system appropriate for each group. IFSCC Magazine. 2003;6:303-7.
2. Kligman AM, Sadiq I, Zhen Y, et al. Experimental studies on the nature of sensitive skin. Skin Res Technol. 2006;12:217-22.
3. Frosch PJ, Kligman AM. A method for appraising the stinging capacity of topically applied substances. J Soc Cosmet Chem. 1977;28:197-209.
4. Ohta M, Hikima R, Ogawa T. Physiological characteristics of sensitive skin classified by stinging test. J Cosmet Sci Soc Jpn. 2000;23:163-7.
5. Berardesca E, Farage M, Mailbach H. Sensitive skin: An overview. Int J Cosm Science. 2013;35:2-8.
6. Chew A, Maibach H. Sensitive skin. In: Loden M, Maibach H, editors. Dry skin and moisturizers: Chemistry and function. CRC Press, Boca Raton: 2000. pp. 429-40.
7. Marriott M, Holmes J, Peters L, et al. The complex problem of sensitive skin. Contact Dermatitis. 2005;53:93-9.
8. Distante F, Bonfigli A, Rigano L, et al. Intra- and inter-individual differences in facial skin biophysical properties. Cosmetic and Toiletries. 2002;7:149-58.
9. Khunger N. Complications. In: Khunger Niti, editor. Step by step chemical peels. 1st ed. New Delhi: Jaypee Brothers Medical Publishers (P) Ltd.; 2009. pp. 280-97.
10. Rajan P, Grimes PE. Skin barrier changes induced by aluminum oxide and sodium chloride microdermabrasion. Dermatol Surg. 2002;28:390-3.
11. Davari P, Gorouhi F, Jafarian S, et al. A randomized investigator-blind trial of different passes of microdermabrasion therapy and their effects on skin biophysical characteristics. Int J Dermatol. 2008;47:508-13.
12. Metelitsa AI, Alster TS. Fractional laser skin resurfacing treatment complications: A review. Dermatol Surg. 2010;36: 299-306.
13. Casey AS, Goldberg D. Guidelines for laser hair removal. J Cosmet Laser Ther. 2008;10:24-33.

14. Gold MH. Lasers and light sources for the removal of unwanted hair. Clin Dermatol. 2007;25:443-53.
15. Bouzari N, Tabatabai H, Abbasi Z, et al. Laser hair removal comparison of long-pulsed Nd:YAG, long-pulsed alexandrite, and long-pulsed diode lasers. Dermatol Surg. 2004;30:498-502.
16. Nanni Ch, Alster TS. Laser-assisted hair removal: Side effects of Q-switched Nd:YAG, long-pulsed ruby, and alexandrite lasers. J Am Acad Dermatol. 1999;41(2 Pt 1):165-71.
17. Ilknur T, Bicak M, Eker P, et al. Effects of the 810-nm diode laser on hair and on the biophysical properties of skin. J Cosmet Laser Ther. 2010;12:269-75.
18. Carruthers J, Carruthers A, Dover JS, et al. Botulinum Toxin. 3rd edn. Saunders: Elsevier; 2013.
19. Carruthers J, Carruthers A, Dover JS, et al. Soft tissue augmentation, 3rd edn. Saunders: Elsevier; 2013.

13
CHAPTER

Skin Care Products for Sensitive Skin: Soaps, Cleansers, and Shampoos

Soumya Jagadeesan, Minu L Mathew

INTRODUCTION

The preceding discussions have elucidated the complexities involved in the care for sensitive skin. The current formulations that are available for sensitive skin are marketed under various loose heterogeneous terms including hypoallergenic, dermatologically tested, for sensitive skin, preservative-free, nonirritating, natural, etc. It is not an uncommon scenario in a dermatology outpatient department for a patient to walk in with a bag full of unsuitable skin care products and a list of ingredients that are taboo. The dermatologist has to perform a tight-rope walk in such a situation, taking into account the patient's skin type, preferences, previous history, and the findings of clinical testing. This chapter discusses the various skin care products that are available for sensitive skin and the principles to be applied while choosing them.

PRINCIPLES IN FORMULATING ANY SKIN-CARE PRODUCT FOR SENSITIVE SKIN

According to Draelos, any sensitive skin product must fulfill certain criteria to be beneficial for this distinctive group of population:[1]
- The known allergens and irritants must be avoided altogether, if not, used in the minimal concentration in the formulation
- As far as possible, the pure form of the material, without contamination should be chosen for formulation. If it is not possible to avoid the contaminant totally, a binding agent can be added for sequestering them

The Sensitive Skin: Treatment Modalities and Cosmeceuticals

- Antioxidants should be employed to prevent the action of auto-oxidation products, which could be responsible for hypersensitivity reactions
- Volatile substances like menthol that could produce cutaneous stimulation should be avoided
- Solvents like polyethylene glycol, which do not penetrate stratum corneum, should be preferred over the solvents that are highly penetrating, like propylene glycol or ethanol
- Surfactants should be chosen wisely; cationic and non-ionic surfactants are preferred over anionic surfactants
- Preservatives like parabens, which have less sensitizing potential, should be chosen over those with a higher sensitizing potential (like formaldehyde).[1]

The products used for sensitive skin may be further improved by adding anti-inflammatory agents, improving barrier function etc. As per the Baumann Skin Typing System, sensitive skin is classified into four types:

- Type 1—the acne type
- Type 2—the flushing rosacea type
- Type 3—the stinging type
- Type 4—sensitive skin, which is often associated with an impaired skin barrier which is susceptible to develop contact dermatitis and irritant dermatitis.

Any ingredient in soaps, shampoos, or other cleansing agents meant for sensitive skin should not induce both visible and invisible signs of sensitivity including acne, flushing, vesiculation, xerosis, edema or stinging, irritation, tightness, itching, and burning. Physiological changes including dehydration, barrier damage, lipid alterations, protein denaturation, stratum corneum swelling, decreased stratum corneocyte adhesion, cytokine release, etc. should also be looked out for.

SOAPS IN SENSITIVE SKIN

The Indian soap industry is a $17 billion industry, including around seven hundred companies with a per capita consumption of 460 g of soap per annum.[2] The primary purpose of soaps have evolved from achieving cleanliness and hygiene benefits to acquiring improved skin tone, moisturization, and fragrance of skin. Ingredients like

Skin Care Products for Sensitive Skin: Soaps, Cleansers, and Shampoos

fragrances, preservatives, and skin-lightening agents added to achieve extra benefits have increased the irritancy of soaps in the form of dry skin, itching, acne, contact dermatitis, and others.[3] Hence mild cleansing bars with milder surfactants devoid of sensitive chemicals, preservatives, and fragrances with a skin friendly pH are preferred, especially in those known to have sensitivity to certain topical skin care products and also in neonates, as their skin barrier function is underdeveloped.[4]

Testing for mildness, therefore, has become one of the priorities of the manufacturing industry. A major step in this direction was the introduction of the "soap-chamber test," where occlusive daily exposure of soaps for 5 days is performed, on the basis of which, soaps are classified as of mild, moderated, and severe irritancy potential. Newer and better *in vitro* and *in vivo* tests have been formulated since then, to calibrate the irritancy potential of the surfactants further; including repeated wash or immersion tests, electrical conductance, transepidermal water loss (TEWL), colorimetry and Doppler velocimetry, and corneosurfametry.[5]

Soap or alkyl carboxylate (sodium laurate) acts as the primary surfactant in majority of the cleansing bars and can produce various cutaneous problems depending upon its pH, length of the fatty acid chain and other secondary components added to it.[4] The most aggressive ones on the skin are the surfactants with C10 to C14 chain lengths. The alkaline nature of the majority of soaps with pH ranging from 9.5 to 11.0 can cause skin damage.[4] Use of milder surfactants like sodium lauryl ether sulphate, sodium cocoyl lauroyl isethionate in syndet bars have shown decreased damage to skin lipids and proteins with reduction in transepidermal loss of water.[6]

Ingredients in skin care and hair care products such as coconut oil and isopropyl myristate may contribute to acne.[7,8] Soaps may also contain various agents that cause sensitivity like unsaturated fatty acids, fragrance mix, coloring agents like red dyes, preservatives like formaldehyde releasing preservatives, parabens, and methyldibromo glutaronitrile.[7-12] Low pH agents like alcohols, which are found in astringents and acids like lactic acid, glycolic acid, and salicylic acid found in soaps are known to produce stinging sensation. Vitamin C in an alcohol base used as a skin-lightening agent in many soaps can produce burning sensation in sensitive individuals.[13]

Methylchloroisothiazolinone and methylisothiazolinone extensively used in soaps and bubble bath are also potential allergens.[14]

Novel techniques using milder surfactants, incorporating humectants and components for enhancing moisturization like oils, occlusive, and emollients, especially in a liquid cleansing formula like shower gels have shown great promise in managing sensitive skin.[15]

SHAMPOOS FOR SENSITIVE SKIN

Shampoos are hair care products in a lather base, used for cleansing hair and scalp on a regular basis and are available in brilliant colors tinged with sweet fragrances. Most of the shampoos contain sodium lauryl sulfate as the active surfactant, which is known to be harsh on skin, causing damage to skin surface proteins and lipids, and increasing TEWL, thereby increasing dryness and itchiness of scalp. A lot of secondary components added to shampoos for added benefits may increase its sensitivity potential as well, causing "scalp sensitivity."

Scalp sensitivity is characterized by presence of vague discomfort in the scalp in the form of burning, stinging, dryness, and rarely trichodynia, which is perceived as an unpleasurable sensation while combing hair.[16] Scalp sensitivity was found to be more intense and frequent in patients with dry, greasy scalps.[17] Frequent shampooing can result in excessive TEWL leading to barrier dysfunction by permitting increased exposure to detergents, and hence forms an important predisposing factor for scalp sensitivity.[18] In a study done by Aleid et al., majority of the patients reported to have scalp sensitivity were females aged between 40 and 59 years with scalp itching or burning sensation being the most common symptoms.[19]

Agents added to increase the moisturizing content of the shampoos to avoid dryness like avocado oil, cocoa butter, coconut oil, and evening primrose oil may aggravate acne in sensitive individuals. Shampoos may contain active coloring agents like red dyes which can induce sensitivity. Stinging sensation in scalp may be aggravated by certain agents in shampoos like eucalyptus oil, alcohol, fragrance, and acids like salicylic acid which are added in shampoos to treat dandruff and seborrheic dermatitis. Certain herbal shampoos claiming to be devoid of allergens may also contain sensitizing substances like aloe vera, chamomile, cucumber, green tea, tea tree oil, etc., which can aggravate scalp sensitivity.[20] Many shampoos marketed as hypoallergenic are found to contain sensitizing agents in the form of botanical extracts and surfactants which are prone to be harsh.

A study done by Zirwas et al. noted that the most common allergens present in shampoos included fragrance (Balsam of Peru, Fragrance Mix 1 & 2), cocamidopropyl betaine (surfactant), methylchloroisothiazolinone/methylisothiazolinone, methyldibromo glutaronitrile/phenoxyethanol, formaldehyde releasers, parabens, iodopropynyl butylcarbamate (preservatives), propyleneglycol (vehicle), benzophenones (structuring agent), and vitamin E.[21] They also found that fragrances were present in almost 95% of the shampoos. Balsam of Peru is a complex substance which contains many potential allergens such as benzoic acid, benzyl acetate, benzyl benzoate, and cinnamic acid, and can be found ubiquitously in hair grooming products, pomade, shampoos, conditioners, shaving lotion, aftershave, perfume, cologne, and cosmetic products with fragrance.[19] Propylene glycol was found in 40% of shampoos sampled in a study and is a common vehicle for topical drugs and cosmetic products.[22] It is a very potent allergen and it is difficult to include a concentration of propylene glycol in a product that does not cause allergy or irritation.[23] Preservatives are used in shampoos and conditioners to prevent contamination and spoilage with bacteria, fungi, yeast, and algae, and many known preservatives like methylchloroisothiazolinone/methylisothiazolinone, methyldibromo glutaronitrile/phenoxyethanol, formaldehyde releasers, parabens, and iodopropynyl butylcarbamate can cause sensitivity and allergic reaction in susceptible individuals.[19]

A study that tested patients' own products found that hair cleansing products including shampoos were the third leading cause of contact dermatitis of the scalp.[23] Patch testing may be required to identify potent allergens in shampoos. Always choose fragrance-free products compared to products labeled as "unscented" as it may contain a masking fragrance.[19] Utmost care has to be taken in choosing a shampoo for a patient with known scalp sensitivity as many shampoos marketed as hypoallergenic may actually contain stinging and sensitizing agents.

CONCLUSION

The formulations used for sensitive skin, ideally are products that have minimum ingredients, absence of sensitizers, minimum number of irritants, and absence of cutaneous sensory and vasodilatory stimulants. They should also reinforce and improve the barrier function. The dermatologists should be well versed with the ingredients that could be used or avoided in this unique subset of population with sensitive skin and advise them accordingly.

REFERENCES

1. Draelos ZD. Sensitive skin: Perceptions, evaluations and treatment. Am J Contact Dermatitis. 1997;8(2):67-78.
2. Indian Soap Industry [Internet]. Indian Soap Industry [cited 2018 June 25]. Available from: http://www.indianmirror.com/indian-industries/soap.html.
3. Abbas S, Goldberg JW, Massaro M. Personal cleanser technology and clinical performance. Dermatol Ther. 2004;17:35.
4. Tyebkhan G. Skin cleansing in neonates and infants—basics of cleansers. Indian J Pediatr. 2002;69:767.
5. Gabard B, Chatelain E, Bieli E, et al. Surfactant irritation: in vitro corneosurfametry and in vivo bioengineering. Skin Res Technol. 2001;7:49.
6. Barel AO, Lambrecht R, Clarys P, et al. A comparative study of the effects on the skin of a classical bar soap and a syndet cleansing bar in normal use conditions and in the soap chamber test. Skin Res Technol. 2001;7:98.
7. Draelos ZD, DiNardo JC. A re-evaluation of the comedogenicity concept. J Am Acad Dermatol. 2006;54:507.
8. Nguyen SH, Dang TP, Maibach HI. Comedogenicity in rabbit: Some cosmetic ingredients/vehicles. Cutan Ocul Toxicol. 2007;26:287.
9. Chatard H. Case of sensitization to perfumes with cutaneous and general reactions. Bull Soc Fr Dermatol Syphiligr. 1957;64:323.
10. Adams RM, Maibach HI. A five-year study of cosmetic reactions. J Am Acad Dermatol. 1985;13:1062.
11. Simpson JR. Dermatitis due to parabens in cosmetic creams. Contact Derm. 1978;5:311.
12. De Groot AC, van Ginkel CJ, Weijland JW. Methyldibromoglutaronitrile (Euxyl K 400): An important "new" allergen in cosmetics. J Am Acad Dermatol. 1996;35:743.
13. Baumann L. Burning and stinging skin (type 3 sensitive skin). In: Baumann L, editor. Cosmetic dermatology, principles and practice. 2nd ed. New York: Mc-Graw Hill; 2009. pp. 133-5.
14. Mowad CM. Methylchloro-isothiazolinone revisited. Am J Contact Dermat. 2000;11:115.

15. Ananthapadmanabhan K, Subramanyan K, Rattinger G. Moisturising cleansers. In: Leyden LJ, Rawlings AV, editors. Skin moisturisation. Cosmetic science technology series. Vol. 25. New York: Marcel Dekker; 2002.
16. Godse K, Zawar V. Sensitive scalp. Int J Trichology. 2012;4:102-4.
17. Farage MA. How do perceptions of sensitive skin differ at different anatomical sites. An epidemiological study? Clin Exp Dermatol. 2009;34:521-30.
18. Misery L, Sibaud V, Ambronati M, et al. Sensitive scalp: Does this condition exist. An epidemiological study? Contact Derm. 2008;58:234-8.
19. Aleid NM, Fertig R, Maddy A, et al. Common allergens identified based on patch test results in patients with suspected contact dermatitis of the scalp. Skin Appendage Disord. 2017;3:7-14.
20. Baumann L. Burning and stinging skin (type 3 sensitive skin). In: Baumann L, editor. Cosmetic dermatology, principles and practice. 2nd edn. New York: Mc-Graw Hill; 2009. pp. 133-35.
21. Zirwas M, Moennich J. Shampoos. Dermatitis. 2009;20:106-10.
22. Lessmann H, Schnuch A, Geier J, et al. Skin-sensitizing and irritant properties of propylene glycol. Contact Derm. 2005;53:247-59.
23. Hillen U, Grabbe S, Uter W. Patch test results in patients with scalp dermatitis: Analysis of data of the Information Network of Departments of Dermatology. Contact Derm. 2007;56:87-93.

14
CHAPTER

Moisturizers in Sensitive Skin

Surabhi Sinha

INTRODUCTION

Sensitive skin can be defined as abnormal subclinical sensory responses to drugs, cosmetics and toiletries, usually in the absence of visible signs of irritation.[1] The complaints commonly associated include itching, burning, stinging, and tightness of the skin. Triggers include cosmetics, drugs and toiletries, plus environmental factors like ultraviolet light, heat, cold, and wind. Different synonyms have been used to describe this entity, including reactive, hyper-reactive, intolerant, and irritable skin. Due to the absence of specific clinical signs, no clear consensual definition has yet been accepted. It is often a self-diagnosed and self-declared condition, without evident clinical traits, and is thus tough to quantify and tougher still to manage!

It usually concerns the face because of its denser nervous network and its great exposure to cosmetic or physical triggering factors. Nevertheless, it is not limited to the face, and sensitive skin may be present on hands or the scalp too.[2] Patients may report feeling dryness or tightness several washing/moisturizing cycles before observable signs of dryness appear.

Sensitive skin may occur in isolation (invisible sensitive skin) or along with specific skin diagnoses such as atopic dermatitis, rosacea, acute contact eczema (visible sensitive skin). The work-up and management should include a complete 2-week discontinuation of any topical application except for synthetic detergent (syndet) bar, clinical examination for underlying dermatoses (rosacea, atopic dermatitis, psoriasis, etc.), a test battery (patch, photopatch, lactic acid stinging test, contact urticaria), and a progressive reintroduction of the cosmetics and skin care products according to a specific protocol.

Such patients may complain of burning/stinging/tingling/itching sensation after application of normally innocuous toiletries or cosmetics. Thus, such patients need an appropriate skin care regime consisting of cleansing, moisturizing, and sun protection with agents that would not contain/contain only minimal amounts of potentially "irritating" ingredients. Here, we seek to delve on the important topic of moisturizers for such patients. Suitable cleansers and therapeutic moisturizers are of benefit as adjuncts to alleviate dryness, restore skin barrier function and reduce susceptibility to irritation in these patients.

A "moisturizer" is an agent designed to make the stratum corneum (SC) soft and more pliant by increasing the hydration of dry skin thus resulting in smoother, suppler and healthier looking skin.[3] They are imperative in patients where there is epidermal barrier alteration, as is present, usually subclinically, in almost all patients of sensitive skin. By restoring the barrier function, covering tiny fissures in the SC and decreasing the transepidermal water loss (TEWL), they improve the skin appearance and elasticity of dry sensitive skin. Water originates in the deeper epidermis and moves upwards by diffusion to hydrate the SC and is eventually lost by evaporation. Most moisturizers in the market nowadays have added ingredients to augment the moisturizing ability.

Products that would benefit the patients would increase skin hydration, mitigate damage to SC proteins, limit damage and stripping of SC lipids, would not contain additives that could augment cutaneous irritation and would optimally deposit lipids, humectants, and cosmetically acceptable occlusive agents that could expedite SC repair.[4-6]

TYPES OF MOISTURIZERS

Occlusives

They form a layer on the skin that is poorly permeated by water. They are especially effective when applied to already dampened skin. Thus, they reduce TEWL. They are the most common type of moisturizers used. However, occlusives have the limitations of odor, greasy feel, and potential allergenicity.

Examples: Petrolatum (prototype), mineral oil/liquid petrolatum, vegetable oil, silicone derivatives, mineral oil, caprylic/capric triglyceride, soybean lipid, beeswax, coconut oil, lanolin, cetyl alcohol, stearyl alcohol.

Humectants

They increase SC hydration by attracting and holding water in the SC (either from dermis or from the environment).

Examples: Glycerin (prototype), ethanolamine or acetamide monoethanolamine (MEA), propylene glycol, ammonium lactate, potassium lactate, sodium lactate, sodium pyrrolidone carboxylic acid (PCA), xylose, hyaluronic acid, sorbitol, urea, polyglycerylmethacrylate, and alpha hydroxyl acids (AHAs)–lactic acid, glycolic acid, tartaric acid.

However, urea and AHAs may cause irritation and stinging on the skin of patients with sensitive skin as they are keratolytic.

Emollients

Materials designed to make the skin feel and appear smooth by filling the spaces between the SC layers with droplets of oil. Some may have additional occlusive properties.

Examples: Mineral oil, cholesterol, squalene, stearic acid, glyceryl stearate, hexyl laureate, soy sterol, lanolin, acetylated lanolin, sunflower (Helianthus annuus) seed oil, wheat germ glycerides.

An ideal moisturizer should be effective, able to restore the lipid barrier and reduce TEWL, cosmetically acceptable, affordable, hypoallergenic, long lasting, and should be rapidly absorbed.[7] For use on the face, they should be nongreasy and noncomedogenic.

Moisturizer Ingredients and Sensitive Skin

The standard components in a conventional oil-in-water over-the-counter facial moisturizer include approximately 80% water, 5% humectants, 4% occlusives/emollients, 6% emulsifiers, 2% silicate, 0.3% thickeners, 0.4% preservatives, and 0.2% fragrance.[8] However,

this is by no means uniform. In addition, nowadays there are further advancements available:
- The ability to deposit specific lipids within SC, e.g., ceramides
- The ability to deposit specific humectants to enhance SC hydration
- The ability to provide occlusivity to reduce TEWL
- Better cosmetic acceptability and better "feel" and "elegance" of products
- Avoidance of ingredients with high propensity of allergic/irritant contact reactions.

Addition of physiologic lipids and humectants or occlusives would benefit patients with sensitive skin. However, they should be present in the correct ratios to be effective and free from adverse effects.

As previously mentioned, the basic function of a moisturizer is to provide hydration to SC. This can be achieved by direct and indirect mechanisms. Direct mechanism is via occlusion and consequent decrease of TEWL (e.g., petrolatum), but the total improvement in skin hydration may not be very significant. Indirect mechanisms include the use of humectants and the incorporation of physiologic lipids that are actively packaged into lamellar bodies in the stratum granulosum and deposited in the upper SC. This is a slower mechanism but the reparative effects on the SC permeability barrier are more prolonged.

Almost half of intercellular lipids in the skin are ceramides, with cholesterol and free fatty acids representing the other constituents. In some individuals with sensitive skin, ceramides 1 and 3 have been believed to be deficient.[9] Draelos and Raymond studied the efficacy of a ceramide-based cream in atopic dermatitis and found significant improvement, both subjectively and objectively.[10] Ceramide based creams use synthetic ceramides that mimic natural ceramides but are contaminant-free and stable. Earlier, bovine sourced ceramides were used and they were associated with higher instances of contamination and contact dermatitis reactions.[11] Ceramides have been shown to improve SC water-holding properties and facilitate barrier repair, imperative in sensitive skin patients.[12,13] They have also been claimed to be an alternative to topical steroids in mild to moderate atopic dermatitis.

Other naturally occurring additives in moisturizers are fatty acid amides such as N-acylethanolamines. Cells naturally produce these substances in order to down-regulate the inflammatory response via cannabinomimetic action on cannabinoid (CB) receptors.[14] Thus, they might have anti-inflammatory, analgesic, and antioxidant properties.[15] The CB1 receptors are found in brain and peripheral tissues, while CB2 receptors are distributed throughout the immune system and in cutaneous nerve fibers.[16] It has been shown that human keratinocytes partake in the peripheral endocannabinoid system.[17]

The most abundant member of this family is palmitoylethanolamide (PEA) or palmitamide MEA, palmitoylethanolamine has been known since the 1950s. It binds to a nuclear receptor peroxisome proliferator-activated receptor alpha (PPAR-α) and potentiates the action of a key endocannabinoid, anandamide, on cannabinoid receptors.[18] The PPAR-α receptor plays a key role in all types of inflammatory responses in the human skin. Rukwied et al. proved that cannabinoid receptor agonists significantly reduced histamine-induced itch and vasodilatation by applying them topically before the administration of histamine.[19] Palmitoylethanolamide has also been demonstrated to decrease mast cell degranulation induced by both neurogenic (substance P) or immune-mediated stimuli.[20,21] It also exerts a potent inhibitory effect on cytokines release from macrophages, and decreases the levels of tumor necrosis factor-α during inflammation and inhibits nitric oxide macrophage production. Also, PEA based moisturizers have been shown to reduce uremic pruritus and itch in atopic dermatitis.[22-24]

Multiple ingredients are used in moisturizers nowadays, some of which are summarized in table 1.

INGREDIENTS TO BE AVOIDED IN MOISTURIZERS FOR SENSITIVE SKIN

Petrolatum is the prototype and the most effective occlusive. However, it may interfere with the SC barrier recovery and hence petrolatum is not the best choice for patients with impaired SC permeability barrier such as in rosacea, atopic dermatitis, and sensitive skin. Similarly, propylene glycol and PCA may rarely produce irritant reactions in patients with sensitive skin. Propylene

Moisturizers in Sensitive Skin

Table 1: Common chemical ingredients used in moisturizers

Chemical compound	Derived from	Function	Used in	Remarks
Glycerin	Natural	Humectant	Moisturizers	–
Petrolatum	Natural	Occlusive, emollient	Moisturizers	–
Ceramides 1–9	One of three lipids of SC	Physiologic lipid, decrease TEWL	Moisturizers	Especially for sensitive skin and atopic dermatitis
Cholesterol	One of three lipids of SC	Emollient, skin conditioner, thickening agent, non-ionic emulsion stabilizer	Moisturizers	–
Cetearyl alcohol	Cetyl alcohol + stearyl alcohol (natural fatty alcohols in coconut oil)	Foam booster, viscosity enhancer, emulsion stabilizer, emollient	Moisturizers, hair conditioners	–
Ceteareth 20	Cetearyl alcohol + ethylene oxide	Emollient, emulsifier	Cosmetics, moisturizers, sunscreens, cleansers	Ethylene oxide and 1,4 dioxane–potential carcinogens, safety concerns
Capric/caprylic triglyceride	Oily liquid from coconut oil	Emollient, occlusive, slippery feel, promotes dispersion of pigment in colored cosmetics	Cosmetics, moisturizers, sunscreens	–
Simethicone/dimethicone	Silicon based polymers	Occlusive, antifoaming, skin protectant, slippery feel, anti-inflammatory	Most skin care products—very safe compound	Decreases redness of rosacea, hence used with more irritating inorganic sunscreen agents

Continued

Continued

Chemical compound	Derived from	Function	Used in	Remarks
Hyaluronic acid	Natural polysaccharide	Humectant (holds 1,000 times water)	Antiaging moisturizers	–
Carbomer	Made from acrylic acid	Emulsifier, holds water and swells	Moisturizers, cosmetics	–
Xanthum gum	Polysaccharide made by fermentation of sucrose by *Xanthomonas campestris*	Holds water and swells, smooth glide, thickener in emulsions	Moisturizers	–
Aloe vera	Natural	Anti-inflammatory	Moisturizers	Improves redness and inflammatory lesions of rosacea
Phytosphingosine	Natural sphingolipid	Antibacterial, anti-inflammatory	Conditioners, moisturizers	–
Sodium lauroyl lactylate	Natural, from sodium salt of lactic acid	Foaming, smooth glide, humectant	Cosmetics, cleansers, moisturizers	–
Methyl/propyl parabens	Paraben	Preservatives	Cosmetics, moisturizers	Allergic reactions known
Phenoxyethanol	Green tea, synthetic also	Preservative	Cosmetics, moisturizers	One of the least irritating preservatives

SC, stratum corneum; TEWL, transepidermal water loss.

glycol is also susceptible to oxidation and may release free radical species, hence may not be ideal in such patients. Alpha hydroxyl acids, urea, alcohol, acetone, and menthol should also be avoided in view of potential irritation. Lanolin can cause allergic and irritant reactions. Fragrances too should be avoided in products meant to be applied over sensitive skin.

CONCLUSION

Management of sensitive skin is fraught with many intricacies. Moisturizers are an integral component of any skin care regime for such patients. It is difficult for sensitive skin patients to discern which product and ingredient benefits their skin and which may lead to an exacerbation of their disease. Thus, as dermatologists it is imperative to know the ingredients of the over-the-counter and prescription products likely to be used by patients so as to guide them.

REFERENCES

1. Kligman AM, Sadiq I, Zhen Y, et al. Experimental studies on the nature of sensitive skin. Skin Res Technol. 2006;12:217-22.
2. Saint-Martory C, Roguedas-Contios AM, Sibaud V, et al. Sensitive skin is not limited to the face. Br J Dermatol. 2008;158:130-3.
3. Loden M. The clinical benefit of moisturizers. J Eur Acad Dermatol Venereol. 2005;19:672-88.
4. Cheong WK. Gentle cleansing and moisturizing for patients with atopic dermatitis and sensitive skin. Am J Clin Dermatol. 2009;10 Suppl.1:13-17.
5. Loden M. Role of topical emollients and moisturizers in the treatment of dry skin barrier disorders. Am J Clin Dermatol. 2003;4:771-8.
6. Buraczewska I, Berne B, Lindberg M, et al. Changes in skin barrier function following long-term treatment with moisturizers, a randomized controlled trial. Br J Dermatol. 2007;156:492-8.
7. Lynde CW. Moisturizers: What they are and how they work. Skin Therapy Lett. 2001;6(13):3-5.
8. Rawlings AV, Canestrari DA, Dobkowski B. Moisturizer technology versus clinical performance. Dermatol Ther. 2004;17:49-56.
9. Di Nardo A, Wertz P, Giannetti A, et al. Ceramide and cholesterol composition of the skin of patients with atopic dermatitis. Acta Derm Venereol. 1998;78(1):27-30.
10. Draelos ZD, Raymond I. The efficacy of a ceramide based cream in mild-to moderate atopic dermatitis. J Clin Aesthet Dermatol. 2018;11(5):30-2.
11. Mizushima H, Fukasawa J, Suzuki T. Phase behavior of artificial stratum corneum lipids containing a synthetic pseudo-ceramide: A study of the function of cholesterol. J Lipid Res. 1996;37(2):361-7.

12. Uchida Y, Holleran WM, Elias PM. On the effects of topical synthetic pseudoceramides: Comparison of possible keratinocyte toxicities provoked by the pseudoceramides, PC104 and BIO391, and natural ceramides. J Dermatol Sci. 2008;51(1):37-43.
13. Park BD, Youm JK, Jeong SK, et al. The characterization of molecular organization of multilamellar emulsions containing pseudoceramide and type III synthetic ceramide. J Invest Dermatol. 2003;121(4):794-801.
14. Noli C, Della Valle MF, Miolo A, et al. Efficacy of ultra-micronized palmitoylethanolamide in canine atopic dermatitis: an open-label multi-centre study. Vet Dermatol. 2015;26(6):432-40, e101.
15. Eberlein B, Eicke C, Reinhardt HW, et al. Adjuvant treatment of atopic eczema: Assessment of an emollient containing N-palmitoylethanolamine (ATOPA study). J Eur Acad Dermatol Venereol. 2008;22(1):73-82.
16. Facci L, Toso RD, Romanello S, et al. Mast cells express a peripheral cannabinoid receptor with differential sensitivity to anandamide and palmitoylethanolamide. Proc Natl Acad Sci USA. 1995;92(8):3376-80.
17. Maccarrone M, Di Rienzo M, Battista N, et al. The endocannabinoid system in human keratinocytes. Evidence that anandamide inhibits epidermal differentiation through CB1 receptor-dependent inhibition of protein kinase C, activating protein-1 and transglutamidase. J Biol Chem. 2003;278:33896-903.
18. Lambert DM, Vandevoorde S, Jonsson KO, et al. The palmitoylethanolamide family: A new class of anti-inflammatory agents? Curr Med Chem. 2002;9:663-74.
19. Rukwied R, Dvorak M, Watkinson A, et al. Putative role of cannabinoids in experimentally induced itch and inflammation in human skin. In: Yosipovitch G, Greaves MW, Fleischer AB Jr, et al., editors. Itch: Basic Mechanisms and Therapy. New York: Marcel Dekker Inc; 2004. p. 115-30.
20. Facci L, Dal Toso R, Romanello S, et al. Mast cells express a peripheral cannabinoid receptor with differential sensitivity to anandamide and palmitoylethanolamide. Proc Natl Acad Sci USA. 1995;92:3376-80.
21. Mazzari S, Canela R, Petrelli L et al. N-(2-hydroxyethyl) hexadecanamide is orally active in reducing edema formation and inflammatory hyperalgesia by down-modulating mast cell activation. Eur J Pharmacol. 1996;300:227-36.
22. Berdyschev EV, Boichot E, Corbel M, et al. Influence of fatty acid ethanolamides and delta 9-tetrahydrocannabinol on cytokine and arachidonate release by mononuclear cells. Eur J Pharmacol. 1997;330:231-40.
23. Berdyshev EV, Boichot E, Corbel M, et al. Effects of cannabinoid receptor ligands on LPS-induced pulmonary inflammation in mice. Life Sci. 1998;63:PL125-29.
24. Costa B, Conti S, Giagnoni G, et al. Therapeutic effect of the endogenous acid amide, palmitoylethanolamide, in rat acute inflammation: inhibition of nitric oxide and cyclo-oxygenase systems. Br J Pharmacol. 2002;137:413-20.

INDEX

Page numbers followed by, *f* refer to figure, and *t* refer to table.

A

Acetamide monoethanolamine 106
Acid mucopolysaccharides 41
Acne 5, 20, 27, 98
    adult onset 19
    development of 20
    pathogenesis of 20
    scars, management of 22
    senile 19
    vulgaris 19, 28
        skin care of 19
Acneiform eruption 41, 41*f*, 43
Alexandrite laser 92
Alkyl carboxylate 99
Allantoin 66
Allergies, seasonal 52
Aloe vera 66, 110
Alpha-adrenergic agonists 46
Alpha-hydroxy acids products 26, 86
Ammonium lactate 106
Androgens, role of 19
Anti-acne medications 22
Anti-acne medications, topical 23
Antibiotic 45
Antioxidants 10*f*
Arcuate pigmentation 44*f*
Asthma 52
Atopy 51
Atrophic facial skin, dermoscopic
    appearance of 44*f*
Atrophy 41, 41*f*, 43
Azelaic acid, topical 35

B

Bacillus olenorium 31
Bacterial lysate 67
Baumann sensitive skin
    classification 20, 21
Benzoic acid 65
Benzophenones 64, 65
Benzoyl peroxide 23, 65
Beta-hydroxy acid 26
    products 86
Bifidobacterium longum extract 67
Body dysmorphic disorder 17
Botulinum toxins 93
Brimonidine, topical 34
Bronopol 64
Burning 9, 21, 98
    sensation 43
Butylparaben 64

C

Calcineurin inhibitor
    topical 45, 54
    use of 54
Camellia sinensis 66
Capacitance 6
Caprylic triglyceride 109
Carbomer 110
Chemical peeling 90
Cholesterol 71, 106, 109
Christensen and Kligman test 62
Cinnamates 64
Cinnamic aldehyde 65

Clarithromycin 36
Cocoyl isethionate 72
Comedones 21
Contact dermatitis 3, 5, 63
    allergic 42, 63, 64
    photoallergic 63, 65
    phototoxic 63, 65
Contact urticaria 59, 63, 65, 105
Corticosteroids, topical 39, 46
Cosmetic intolerance syndrome 57, 58, 60
    management of 58
Crisaborole 16
Cyclomethicone 27

D

Dehydration 98
Demodex folliculorum 31, 42
Demodex mite 32, 33
Dermatitis 39, 52
    atopic 2, 5, 49, 52, 54
    perioral 42, 42*f*, 45*f*, 46*f*
    rosaciformis steroidica 39
    skin care in 49
Dermis 70
Dermo-epidermal junction 70
Diazolidinyl urea 64
Dibenzoylmethane 64, 65
Diethyltoluamide 65
Dimethicone 109
Dimethyl sulfoxide 62, 65
Dimethyloldimethyl 64
Diode laser 92
DMSO test 62
Doxycycline 25, 35
Dry skin 2, 84
    care of 80

E

Eczema, atopic 52
Edema 32, 98
Electrolyte homeostasis 69
Embryonic endoderm 5
Emollients, role of 73
Endothelin receptors 51

Epidermis 70
Erythema 3*f*, 9, 40, 54, 92
Erythematotelangiectatic rosacea 33
Ethanolamine 106
Ethylparaben 64
Eyelid margins 33

F

Facial sting testing 59
Fatty acids
    saturated 74
    unsaturated 74
Flavonoids 10*f*
Follicular
    epithelium 21, 41
    hyperkeratinization 20
Formaldehyde 64, 65, 98
Free fatty acids 51

G

Gentle skin care 34
Ginkgo biloba 66
Glycemic index 28
Glycerin 109
Glyceryl stearate 106
Glyceryl thioglycolate 64
Glycolic acid 106
Glycyrrhiza inflata 75
Gnathophyma 32

H

Hair 70
    follicles 33
    removal lasers 92
Helianthus annuus 106
Helicobacter pylori 32
Hirsutism 42
Hordeolum 32
Hormonal influences 61
Hormones 83
Hyaluronic acid 106, 110
Hydantoin 64
Hydrocarbons 73
Hydrochloric acid 65
Hydroxy acids 16

Index

Hyperpigmentation 42
Hypersensivity 31
Hypertrichosis 43, 44*f*
Hypoallergenic cosmetics 58
Hypopigmentation 42

I

Imidazolidinyl urea 64
Intense pulsed light 92
Isotretinoin 25, 36
Itching 9, 21, 98

K

Koebner response,
    development of 55

L

Lactic acid 9, 32, 106
  facial sting test 62
  stinging test 105
Lanolin 64
Lasers
  assisted hair removal 92
  fractional
    ablative 26
    resurfacing 91
Light and laser therapy 36
Linoleic acid 74
Linolenic acid 74

M

Macrolides 36
Malassezia furfur 75
Massage, role of 74
Menthol 65
Methylchloroisothiazolinone 100
Methyldibromo glutaronitrile 64
Methylisothiazolinone 100
Methylparaben 64, 110
Metophyma 32
Metronidazole, topical 35
Microdermabrasion 91
Minocycline 25, 35
Moisturizers 62, 86, 104
  role of 73
  types of 105
Morbihan disease 32
Muizzuddin classification 14

N

Neodymium-doped yttrium
    aluminum garnet 26, 91, 92
Nicotinic acid 3
Nitric oxide, role of 40
Noxious pain receptors 51

O

Ocular irritation 31
Ocular rosacea 33
Oleic acid 74
Oral medications 25
Oxymetazoline, topical 35

P

Papulopustular lesions 41
Papulopustular rosacea 33
Para-aminobenzoic acid 65
Parabens 65
Patch 105
  tests 59
Perifollicular hypopigmentation 44*f*
Peroxisome proliferator-activated
    receptor alpha 108
Phenoxyethanol 110
Phosphoric acid 65
Photopatch 105
  tests 59
Photosensitivity 42
Phymatous rosacea 33
Phytosphingosine 110
Pimples 21
Platelet-rich plasma 35
Polyethylene glycol 65
Polyglycerylmethacrylate 106
Polygonal vessels 44*f*
Pons-Guiraud classification 14
Potassium
  lactate 106

titanyl phosphate 36
Powder facial foundation 15
P-phenylenediamine 64
Propionibacterium acnes 21, 23
Propylene glycol 64, 65, 106
Propylparaben 64, 110
Protein denaturation 98
Psoriasis 2, 5, 49, 53, 55, 105
Pustules 31

R

Radiation 69
Red skin syndrome 39
Retinaldehyde 23
Retinoic acid 23, 32
Retinoids, topical 23
Rhinophyma 31, 32
Rosacea 2, 3, 4f, 5, 31, 35, 42, 42f, 51, 104
   consensus guidelines 34
   cutaneous 33
   sensitive skin of 31, 34
   steroid induced 39
Ruby laser 92

S

Salicylic acid 65, 76
Scalp, care of 75
Sebaceous hyperplasia 32
Seborrhea 19
Seborrheic dermatitis 2, 3, 5, 49, 51, 52
Sensitive skin 1, 2, 4, 4f, 6, 14, 19, 20, 22f, 49, 55, 60, 61, 62t, 63, 66, 82, 84, 85, 89, 92, 94, 97, 104, 106, 108
   care of 14, 69
   classifications of 83t
   diagnosis of 9
   instructions for
     cosmetic use for 87
     makeup use for 87
   invisible 3, 104
   management of 111

pathophysiology of 50
role of 20
shampoos for 100
skin care product for 97
soaps in 98
syndrome 15, 17
treatment of 62, 67
triggers for 7t
visible 3, 3f, 104
Silicone derivatives 106
Simethicone 109
Skin 69
   adult 69, 70, 70t
   barrier dysfunction 75
   behavior 84
   care 31, 78, 79
     products 97
     routine 22, 26
   disorders 83
   fragility 16
   immune system 40
   injuries, prevention of 80
   irritable 14
   neonatal 69, 70, 70t, 76
   normal 84
   oily 84
   sensitivity 32
   structure 70
   thickening of 31
   type determination 84, 84t
   types of 82, 84
Soap-chamber test 99
Sodium
   chloride 91
   hydroxide 65
   lactate 106
   laurate 99
   lauryl lactylate 110
   lauryl sulphate 72
     occlusion test 62
   pyrrolidone carboxylic acid 106
   salicylate 16
Soft tissue fillers 94
Sorbic acid 65
Sorbitol 106

Index

Staphylococcus epidermidis 32
Status cosmeticus 43, 54, 57
Stearic acid 106
Steroid
  abuse
    chronic 41*f*, 43*f*, 45*f*
    topical 44*f*
  damaged, topical 39, 41*f*, 43
  topical 55
Stratum corneum 7, 63, 105, 110
  hydration 51
  swelling 98
Stress 83
  psychological 61
Sun protection 34
Sunscreen 64, 86
  inorganic 66
Sweat glands 70

T

Tacrolimus, topical 46*f*
Tartaric acid 106
Telangiectasia 31, 41, 41*f*, 43
Tetracyclines 25, 35
Thermoregulation 69
Tinea incognito 42, 43*f*
Toluene sulphonamide 64
Topical steroid damaged/dependent face, management of 43
Tortuous vessels 44*f*

Transepidermal water loss 6, 20, 49, 71, 80, 91, 105, 110
Transretinoic acid 23
Tretinoin 23
Tumor necrosis factors alpha 9

U

Ultraviolet
  light and heat 31
  radiation 82
Urticaria, development of 65

V

Vascular system 70
Vernix caseosa 71
  role of 71
Vesiculation 98
Vulvar erythema 50

W

Wheat germ glycerides 106

X

Xanthum gum 110
Xerosis 98
Xylose 106

Z

Zinc oxide 75

www.ingramcontent.com/pod-product-compliance
Ingram Content Group UK Ltd
Pitfield, Milton Keynes, MK11 3LW, UK
UKHW061222180426
11947UKWH00026B/1964